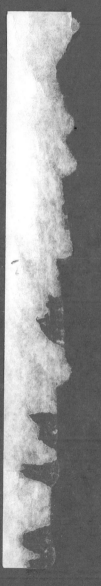

the
Beauty book

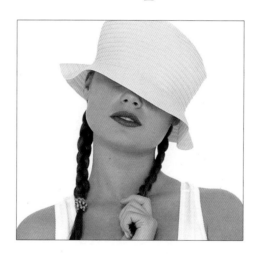

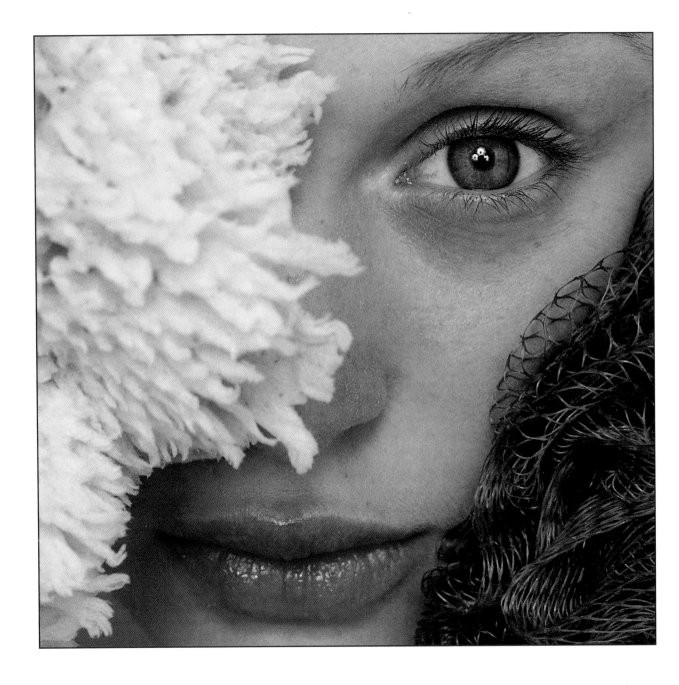

the Beauty book

super skin, perfect hair, luscious lips, fabulous nails

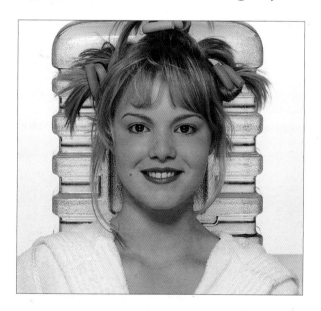

Sally Norton and Jacki Wadeson

LORENZ BOOKS

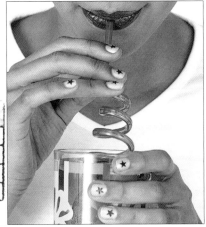

First published in 1999 by Lorenz Books

Lorenz Books is an imprint of
Anness Publishing Limited
Hermes House
88–89 Blackfriars Road
London SE1 8HA

© Anness Publishing Limited 1999

A CIP catalogue record for this book is available from the British Library

ISBN 0 7548 0257 4

Publisher Joanna Lorenz
Project Editors Sarah Ainley and Cathy Marriott
Designers Siân Keogh and Ian Sandom
Jacket Design Anne Fisher
Photography Nick Cole and Alistair Hughes
Indexer Vicki Robinson

Skincare and *Make-up* hair and make-up by Debbi Finlow; *Haircare* hair by Kathleen Bray
assisted by Wendy M.B. Cook, make-up by Vanessa Haines;
Nailcare hair and make-up by Sue Moxley

Previously published in four separate volumes, *Instant Skincare*, *Instant Haircare*, *Instant Make-up* and *Instant Nailcare*

Printed and bound in Singapore

1 3 5 7 9 10 8 6 4 2

Contents

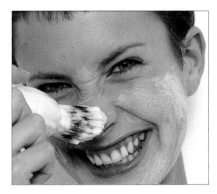 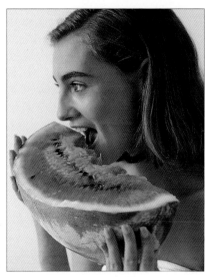 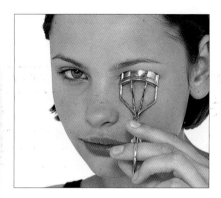

Introduction

If you are interested in your looks and in making the most of them, then this is the book for you. The secret to looking good is knowing your individual beauty needs – how to create a beauty regime that works for you and how to deal with your particular beauty problems. This book will help you master the basics of skincare, haircare, make-up, nailcare, diet and exercise, to get you in tiptop condition and on track for a healthy lifestyle, and is full of advice, tips and tricks of the trade for professional results at a fraction of the cost. In no time at all, you'll be feeling fantastic and looking better than ever!

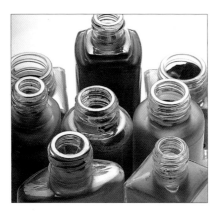

Above: The wonderful world of make-up awaits between the pages of this book…

Right: Everyone has different beauty needs but we all enjoy a bit of pampering.

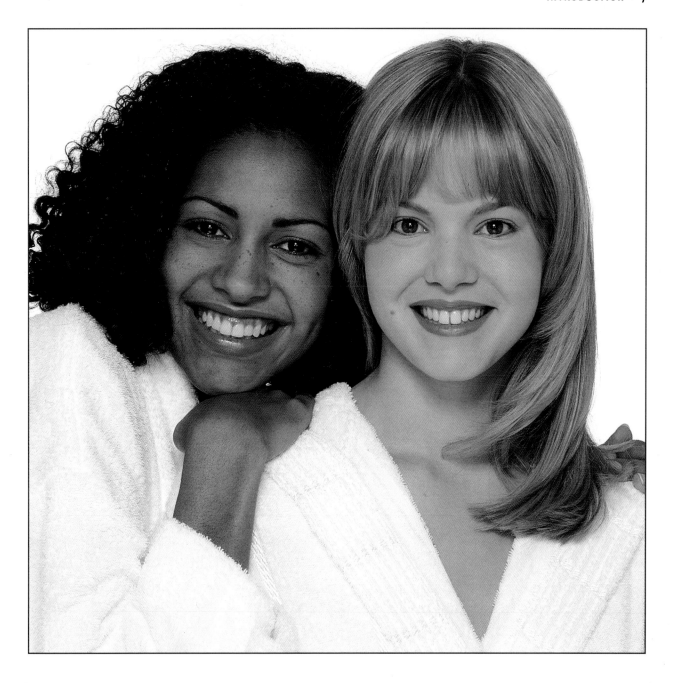

Beautiful Skin

Clear, soft and supple skin is one of the greatest beauty assets. While your actual skin type is determined by your genes, there's plenty you can do on a day-to-day basis to ensure it always looks as good as possible. Understanding how your skin functions will awaken you to its special needs. In this book we'll show you how to care for your own specific skin type. You can't neglect your complexion for months or years, then make up for it with expensive and intensive attention in the short term. You'll reap the benefits by regularly spending time and care on your skin. It's never too early or too late to follow a good skincare regime – because the results will last a lifetime.

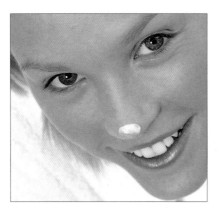

Above: Moisturizing your skin every day keeps it healthy and glowing.

Right: Remember to look after the skin on your whole body for all over beauty.

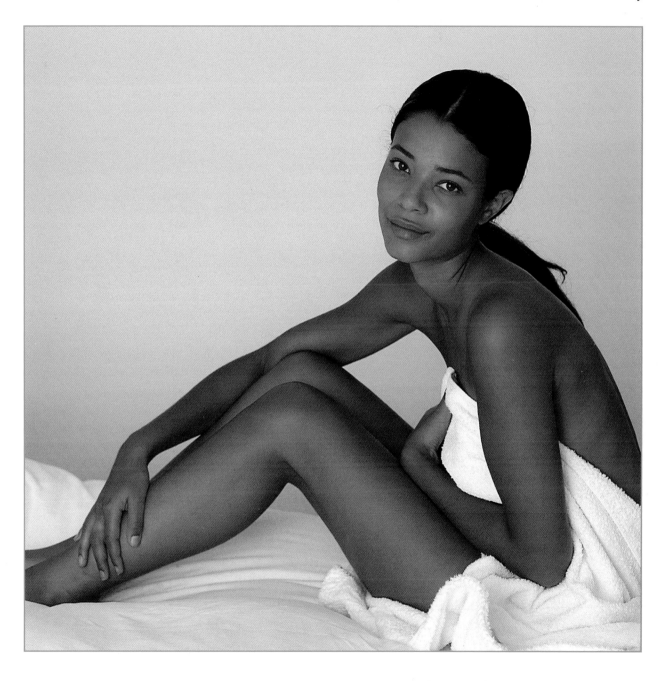

What is Skin?

Skin is your body's largest organ. Every woman can have beautiful skin no matter what her age, race or colouring. The secret is to understand how your skin functions and to treat it correctly. Your skin is made up of two main layers, called the epidermis and the dermis.

The epidermis

This is the top layer of skin and the one you can actually see. It protects your body from invasion and infection and helps to seal in moisture. It's built up of several layers of living cells that are then topped by sheets of dead cells. It's constantly growing, with new cells being produced at its base. They quickly die and are pushed up to the surface by the arrival of new ones. These dead cells eventually flake away, which means that every new layer of skin provides another chance to have a glowing complexion.

The lower levels of living cells are fed by the blood supply from underneath, whereas the upper dead cells only need water to ensure they are kept really plump and smooth.

The epidermis is responsible for your colouring, as it holds the skin's pigment. Its thickness varies from area to area – e.g. it's much thicker on the soles of your feet than on your eyelids.

The dermis

The dermis is the layer that lies underneath the epidermis, and it is composed entirely of living cells. It consists of bundles of tough fibres that give your skin its elasticity, firmness and strength. There are also blood vessels, which feed vital nutrients to these areas.

Whereas the epidermis can usually repair itself and make itself as good as new, the dermis will be permanently damaged by injury. The dermis also contains the following specialized organs:

Sebaceous glands

These tiny organs usually open into hair follicles on the surface of your skin. They produce an oily secretion, called sebum, which is your skin's natural lubricant.

The sebaceous glands are concentrated mostly on the scalp and face – particularly around the nose, cheeks, chin and forehead, which is why these are usually the most oily areas of your skin. The oily areas across the forehead and down the nose and chin are called the T-zone.

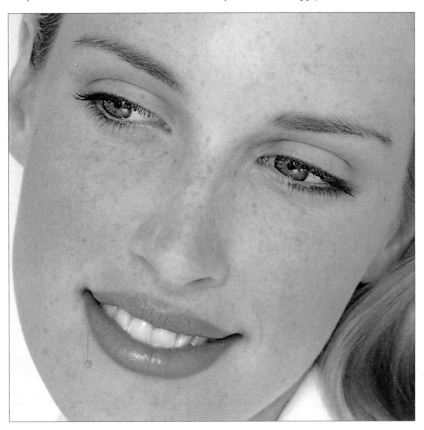

Left: Understanding your skin in the way a beautician would allows you to give it the care it deserves and to appreciate why certain factors are good for it – and others are not.

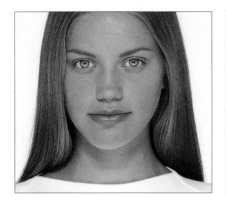

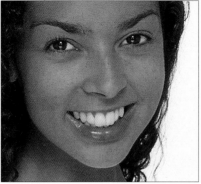

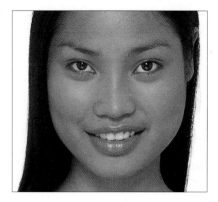

Above: Your skin is a sensor of pain, touch and temperature, offering protection to your inner body and a means of eliminating waste.

Above: Your skin can cleanse, heal and even renew itself. How effectively it does these things is partly governed by how you care for it.

Above: Skin is a barometer of your emotions. It becomes red when you're embarrassed and quickly begins to show the signs of stress.

Sweat glands

There are millions of sweat glands all over your body, and their main function is to regulate your body temperature. When sweat evaporates on the skin's surface, the temperature of your skin drops.

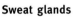

Hairs

Hairs grow from hair follicles. They can help keep your body warm by trapping air underneath them.

THE MAIN FUNCTIONS OF YOUR SKIN

■ It acts as a thermostat, retaining heat or cooling you down with sweat.

■ It offers protection from potentially harmful things.

■ It acts as a waste disposal. Certain waste is expelled from your body 24 hours a day through your skin.

■ It provides you with a sense of touch.

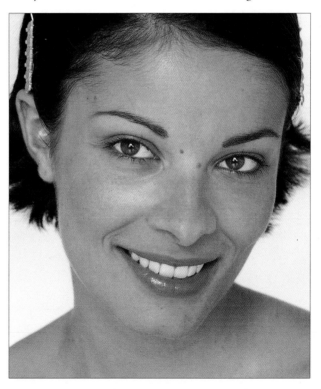

Left: The condition of your skin is an overall sign of your health. It reveals stress, a poor diet and a lack of sleep. Taking care of your health will benefit your skin.

What's your Skin Type?

There's no point spending a fortune on expensive skincare products if you buy the wrong ones for your skin type.

The key to developing a skincare regime that works for you is to analyze your skin type first.

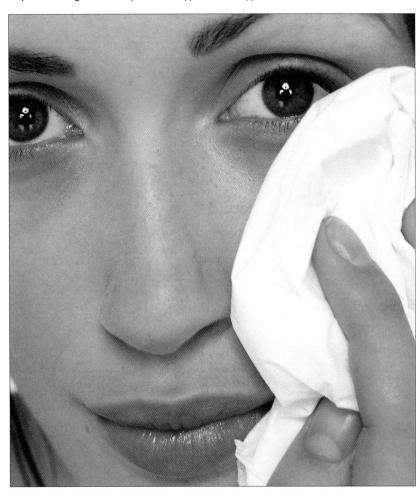

Above: You know best how your skin reacts to different things so check your skin type before you buy lots of skincare products. Even if you've been told what your skin type is at some stage, it is a good idea to run through this quiz now as your skin will change over a period of time.

SKINCARE QUIZ

To develop a better understanding of your skin and what skincare routine and products will suit it best, start by answering the questions here. Then add up your score and check the list at the end to discover which of the skin types you fit into. Remember that your skin type can change over time — try to do this skincare quiz each year to check that you are still using the right skincare products and following the best skincare routine.

1 How does your skin feel if you cleanse it with facial wash (soap) and water?
A Tight, as though it's too small for my face.
B Smooth and comfortable.
C Dry and itchy in places.
D Fine – quite comfortable.
E Dry in some areas and smooth in others.

2 How does your skin feel if you cleanse it with cream cleanser?
A Relatively comfortable.
B Smooth and comfortable.
C Sometimes comfortable, sometimes itchy.
D Quite oily.
E Oily in some areas and smooth in others.

3 How does your skin usually look by midday?
A Flaky patches appearing.
B Fresh and clean.
C Flaky patches and some redness.
D Shiny.
E Shiny in the T-zone.

4 How often do you break out in spots?
A Hardly ever.
B Occasionally, perhaps before or during your period.
C Occasionally.
D Often.
E Often – in the T-zone.

5 How does your skin react when you use facial toner?
A It stings.
B No problems.
C Stings and itches.
D Feels fresher.
E Feels fresher in some areas but stings in others.

6 How does your skin react to a rich night cream?
A It feels very comfortable.
B Comfortable.
C Sometimes feels comfortable, other times feels irritated.
D Makes my skin feel very oily.
E Oily in the T-zone, and comfortable on the cheeks.

Now add up the number of As, Bs, Cs, Ds and Es. Your skin type is the one which has the majority of answers. You are now ready to follow the right skincare routine for your skin type.
Mostly As: Your skin is DRY.
Mostly Bs: Your skin is NORMAL.
Mostly Cs: Your skin is SENSITIVE.
Mostly Ds: Your skin is OILY.
Mostly Es: Your skin is COMBINATION.

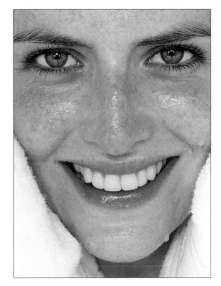

Above: Is traditional soap and water cleansing right for you?

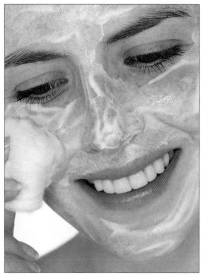

Above: Or is the gentle touch of a cleansing cream a softer option?

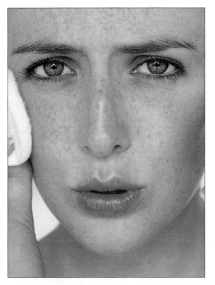

Above: Does using a facial toner make your skin sting?

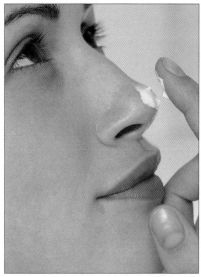

Above: Are your face creams an embarrassment of riches?

The Top Skincare Products

Before you can devise the best regime for yourself and give your skin some special care, you need to understand what the main skincare products are designed to do. From a basic soap and water cleansing routine, today's skincare ranges have evolved into a sophisticated selection.

Facial washes

These scrubs are designed to be lathered up with water to dissolve grime, dirt and stale make-up from the skin's surface.

Cleansing bars

A wash to cleanse your skin without stripping it of moisture – ordinary soap is too drying for most skins. They're refreshing for oilier skin types and help keep pores clear and prevent pimples.

Cream cleansers

These light creams are a wonderful way to cleanse drier complexions. They generally have quite a light, fluid consistency to make them easy to spread onto the skin. They contain oils to dissolve surface dirt and make-up, so they can be easily swept from your skin with cotton wool (cotton balls). Use damp cotton wool if you prefer a fresher finish.

Toners and astringents

Designed to refresh and cool your skin, toners quickly evaporate after being applied to the skin with cotton wool (cotton balls). They can also remove excess oil from the surface layers of your skin. The word "astringent" on the bottle means it has a higher alcohol content and is only suitable for oily skins. The words "tonic" and "toner" mean that they're useful for normal or combination skins, as they are gentler. Those with dry and sensitive skins should usually avoid these products, as they can be too drying. Generally, if the product stings your face, move onto a gentler formulation or weaken it by adding a few drops of distilled water (available from a pharmacist).

Moisturizers

These creams form a barrier film on the surface of your skin and prevent moisture loss from the top layers. This makes the skin feel softer and smoother. Generally, the drier your skin the thicker the moisturizer you should choose. All skin types need a moisturizer.

Moisturizers today also contain a myriad of other ingredients to treat your skin. The most valuable one to look for is an ultraviolet (UV) filter. With this, your moisturizer will give your skin year-round protection from the ageing and burning rays of the sun.

Eye make-up removers

When ordinary cleansers aren't sufficient to remove stubborn eye make-up, use a special make-up remover. If you wear waterproof mascara check that the product you use is designed to remove it.

Night creams

These are thick creams designed to give your skin extra moisturizing and pampering while you sleep.

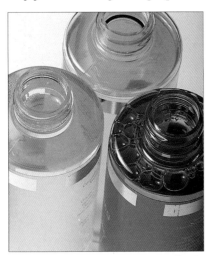

Above: Put some zing into your skincare regime with a refreshing toner or astringent treatment.

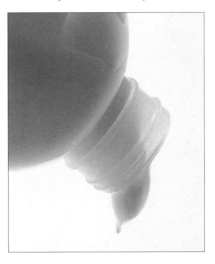

Above: Creamy cleansers should be a top priority for drier complexions, as they cleanse and nourish at the same time.

Right: Before you make up a skincare regime for yourself, you need to know the key benefits of each product.

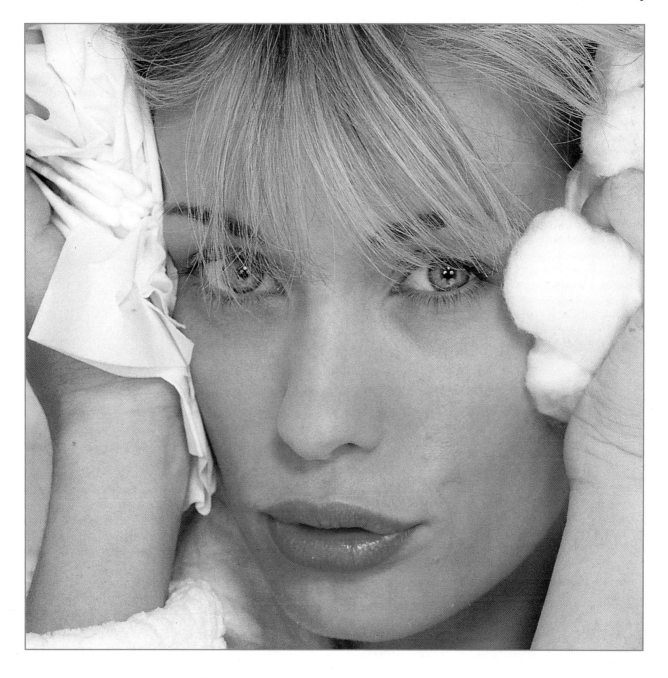

The Perfect Skincare Routine

Skincare can be confusing these days because there are so many products around. Basically, your skin needs two staples: cleanser and moisturizer. Other products – toner, exfoliator, and eye cream or gel – are extras. If you are using more than three or four products daily and your skin keeps breaking out or reacting, you may be trying too hard. Simplify your routine (it should not take more than 10 minutes to do twice a day), and use basic formulas. You really will be amazed by the speed at which your skin improves.

Cleanse

Use water-soluble emulsions (creams) or gels with tepid (not hot) water or wipe-off lotions. If your skin is oily, use pH-balanced soap-free bars. Splash your face with water – it will instantly give your skin a better tone.

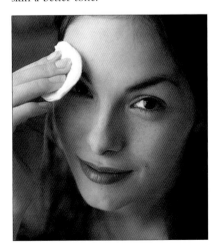

Above: Toners improve skin texture. Apply to oily skin after cleansing.

Tone

If you want to tone, buy alcohol-free toner or use rosewater to freshen your skin. If your skin is dry and you have been using toner, stop and it will instantly improve.

Moisturize

Ideally, use water-based creams and emulsions; if your skin frequently breaks out in pimples and blackheads, try a lighter, oil-free moisturizer.

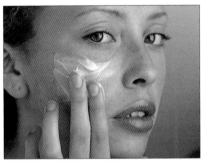

Above: Use upward and outward strokes to apply moisturizer.

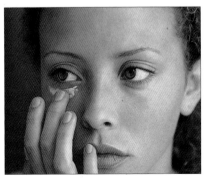

Above: Pat under-eye creams, gels and face creams on with your fingertips.

Exfoliate

Do this once a week only. Too much buffing will overstimulate and irritate your skin. Fine-grained exfoliators remove dead skin cells and instantly soften your skin.

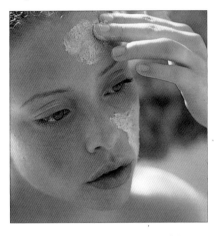

Above and below: Fine-grained exfoliators should be massaged gently into the skin and then rinsed away thoroughly.

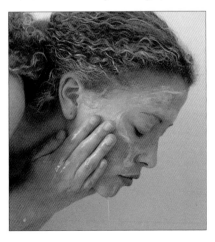

Mask

Simple mud- and clay-based cleansing masks are messy but effective. Rich cold creams make good moisturizing masks for dry or sun-exposed skin: smother your skin with the cream, let the skin absorb as much of the cream as possible and wipe off the excess with soft tissue.

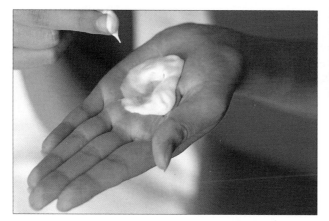

1 Put some of the mask into your hand first.

Then stroke it over clean, exfoliated skin, avoiding the eye area. (**2**)

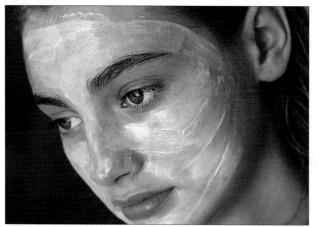

3 Relax for at least 10 minutes.

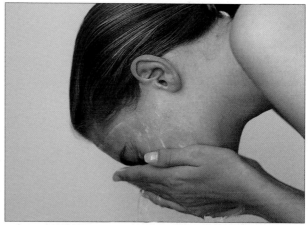

4 Rinse the face mask off thoroughly with tepid or warm water.

Maintaining Normal Skin

This is the perfect, balanced skin type. It has a healthy glow, with a fine texture and no open pores. It rarely develops spots or shiny areas. In fact, it's quite rare to find a normal skin, especially as all skins tend to become slightly drier as you get older.

SPECIAL CARE FOR NORMAL SKIN

Your main concern is to keep normal skin functioning well and, as a result of this, to let it continue the good job it's already doing. It naturally has a good balance of oil and moisture levels. Your routine should include gently cleansing your skin to ensure that surface grime and stale make-up are removed, and to prevent a build-up of sebum. Then you should boost moisture levels with moisturizer, to protect your skin and ensure its moisture content is balanced.

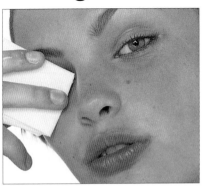

1 Eye make-up should always be removed carefully. Going to bed with mascara on can lead to sore, puffy eyes. Applying new make-up on the top of stale make-up is positively unhygienic too. Choose your product according to whether you're wearing ordinary or waterproof mascara.

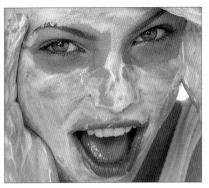

2 Splash your face with water, then massage in a gentle facial wash and work it up to a lather for about 30 seconds. Take this opportunity to lightly massage your face, as this will boost the supply of blood to the surface of your skin – which will result in a rosier complexion.

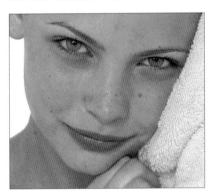

3 Rinse with clear water, then pat your face with a soft towel to absorb residual water from the surface of your skin. Don't rub at your skin, especially around the eyes, as this can encourage wrinkling.

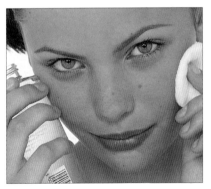

4 Cool your skin with a freshening toner. Again, be careful to avoid the delicate eye area as this can become more prone to dryness.

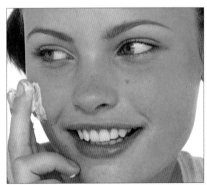

5 Dot moisturizer onto your face, then massage it in with your fingertips using light, gentle upward strokes. This will leave a protective film on the skin and allow make-up to be easily applied.

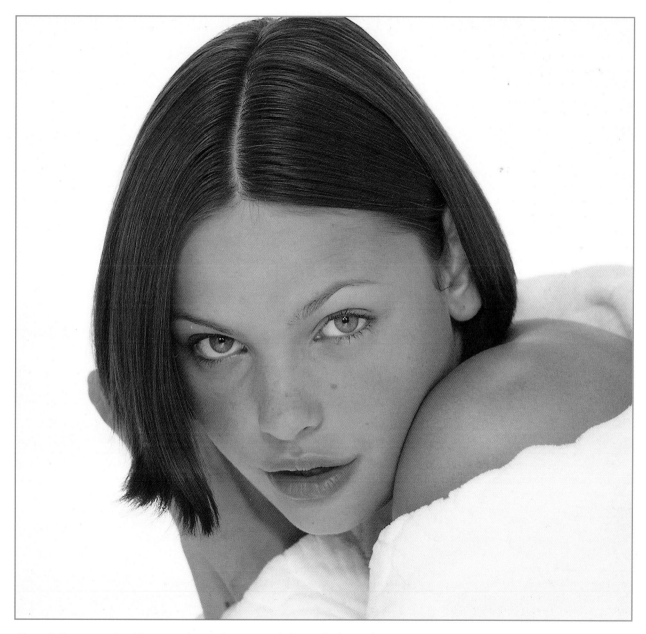

Above: Follow a regular skincare regime to keep normal skin as fresh as a daisy.

The Fresh Approach to Oily Skin

This skin type usually has open pores and an oily surface, with a tendency towards pimples, blackheads and a sallow appearance. This is due to the overproduction of sebum. Unfortunately, this skin type is the one most prone to acne. The good news is that this oiliness will make your skin stay younger-looking for longer – so there are some benefits!

SPECIAL CARE FOR OILY SKIN

It's important not to treat oily skin too harshly, although this can be tempting when you're faced with a fresh outbreak of pimples. Overenthusiastic treatment can encourage the oil glands to produce even more sebum, whilst it will leave the surface layers dry and dehydrated.

The best way to care for oily skin is to use products that gently cleanse away oils from the surface and unblock pores, without drying out and damaging it. The visible part of your skin actually needs water, not oil, to stay soft and supple.

ACNE ALERT

Anyone who has acne knows what a distressing condition it is. As well as being a problem that runs in families, it's thought to be triggered by a change in hormones during adolescence, which results in more sebum being produced by your skin. It can also be aggravated by stress, poor lifestyle and poor skincare.

Careful skincare will help keep acne under control. Avoid picking at pimples, as this can lead to scarring. Try over-the-counter blemish treatments. Today's formulations contain ingredients that are very successful at treating this problem. Products containing tea tree oil can be very effective. If these aren't successful, consult your doctor who may be able to provide treatment or refer you to a specialist dermatologist.

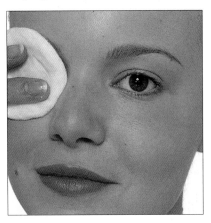 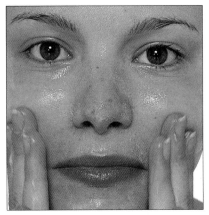 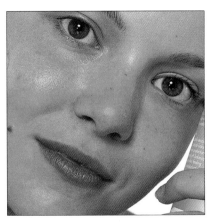

1 Even though the remainder of your face is prone to oiliness, always remember that the skin around your eyes is very delicate. Soak a cotton wool (cotton ball) pad with a non-oily remover and hold it over your eyes for a few seconds to give it time to dissolve the make-up. Then lightly stroke away the mascara and make-up from the eyelids and your upper and lower lashes.

2 Splash your face with tepid water, then lather up with a gentle foaming facial wash. This is a better choice than ordinary soap, as it won't strip away moisture from your skin, but it will remove the grime, dirt and oil that accumulates during the day. Massage gently over damp skin with your fingertips, then carefully rinse away with lots of warm water.

3 Soak a cotton wool (cotton ball) pad with a refreshing astringent lotion. Sweep it over your skin to refresh and cool it. This liquid should not irritate or sting your skin – if it does, swap to a product with a gentler formulation or dilute your existing one with some distilled water (available from a pharmacist). Continue until the cotton wool comes up completely clean.

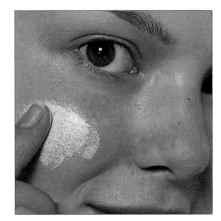

4 Even oily skin needs a gentle moisturizer, because a moisturizer helps to seal water into the top layers of the skin to keep your face soft and supple. Choose a light, watery fluid rather than a heavy formulation, as this will be enough for you.

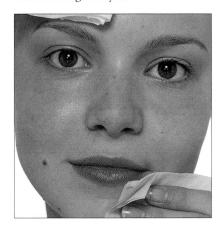

5 Allow the moisturizer to sink into your skin for a few minutes, then press a clean tissue over your face to absorb the excess and to prevent a shiny complexion.

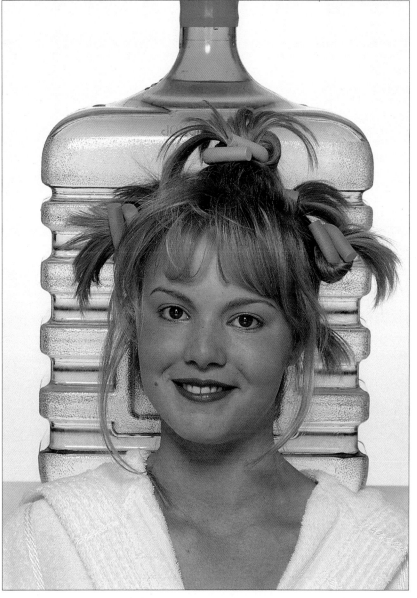

Above: Boosting your skin's moisture levels and controlling excess oiliness will ensure a beautifully clear complexion.

Nourishing Care for Dry Skin

If your skin tends to feel one size too small, it's a fair bet you've got a dry complexion. It's caused by too little sebum in the lower levels of the skin and too little moisture in the upper levels. It can feel tight after washing. At its worst, it can be flaky, with flakiness in your eyebrows, and have a tendency to promote premature ageing with the emergence of fine lines and wrinkles.

SPECIAL CARE FOR DRY SKIN

The condition of dry skin can be aggravated by overuse of soap, detergents and toners. It is also affected by exposure to hot sun, cold winds and central heating. Opt for the gentle approach, concentrating on boosting the skin's moisture level to plump out fine lines and make it soft and supple.

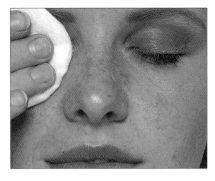

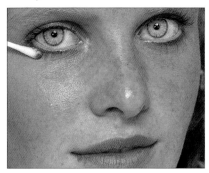

1 Pour a little oil-based eye make-up remover onto a cotton wool (cotton ball) pad and sweep it over the eye area. This oily product will also help soothe dryness in the delicate eye area, but a little goes a long way. If you overload the skin here with an oily product it can cause puffiness and irritation.

2 Clean up stubborn flecks with a cotton bud (swab) dipped in eye make-up remover. Be careful not to get the remover in your eyes but work as closely as you can to the eyelashes to remove all signs of make-up.

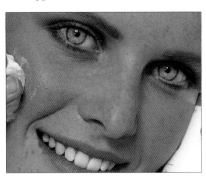

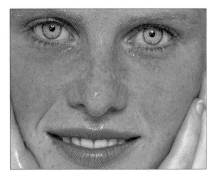

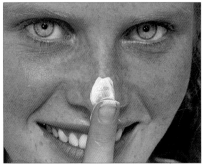

3 Choose a creamy cleanser that will melt away dirt and make-up from the surface of your skin. Leave the cleanser on for a few moments for it to work, before sweeping it away with a cotton wool (cotton ball) pad. Use gentle upward movements to prevent stretching the skin and encouraging lines.

4 Many women with dry skins say that they miss the feeling of water on their skin. However, you can splash your face with cool water to remove excess cleanser and to refresh your skin. This will also help boost the blood circulation in your face, which means a brighter complexion.

5 This is the most important step of all for dry skins – a nourishing cream to seal moisture into the upper levels of your skin. Opt for a thick cream, rather than a runny lotion, as this contains more oil than water. Give the moisturizer a few minutes to sink into your skin before applying make-up.

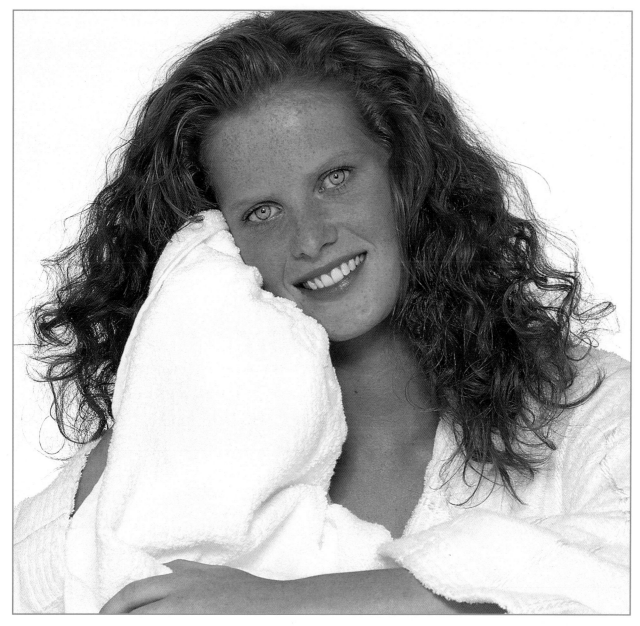

Above: Nourish dry skin by using a thick moisturizer to keep it as soft and supple as possible.

Balanced Care for Combination Skin

Combination skin needs careful attention because it has a blend of oily and dry patches. The centre panel, or T-zone, across the forehead and down the nose and chin tends to be oily and needs to be treated like oily skin. However, the other areas are prone to dryness and flakiness due to lack of moisture and need to be treated like dry skin. Having said this, some combination skins don't follow the T-zone pattern and can have patches of dry and oily skin in other arrangements. If you're unsure of your skin's oily and dry areas, press a tissue to your face an hour after washing it. Any greasy patches on the tissue signify oily areas — this will enable you to develop a routine appropriate for your skin.

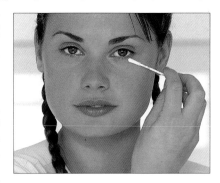

1 Choose an oil-based eye make-up remover to clear away every trace of eye make-up from this delicate area, which is prone to dryness. Use a cotton bud (swab) to remove any stubborn traces. Splash with cool water afterwards to rinse away any excess oil.

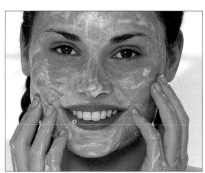

2 Use a foaming facial wash in the morning to cleanse your skin. This will ensure the oily areas are clean and that the pores on your nose are kept clear. Massage a little onto damp skin, concentrating on the oily areas. Leave for a few seconds to dissolve the dirt, then rinse.

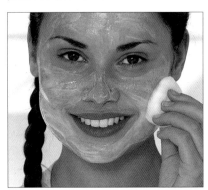

3 In the evening, switch to a cream cleanser, to ensure the dry areas of your skin are kept clean and soothed on a daily basis. This will give you a balance between excess oiliness or dryness. Massage well into your skin, concentrating on the drier areas, then remove with cotton wool pads (cotton balls).

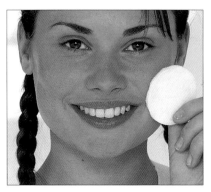

4 To freshen your skin, you need to use two different strengths of toners. Choose a stronger astringent for the oily areas, and a mild skin freshener for the drier ones. This isn't as expensive as you think, because you'll only need to use a little of each. Sweep over your skin with cotton wool pads (cotton balls).

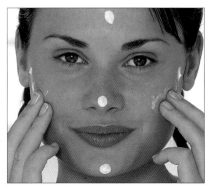

5 Smooth moisturizer onto your entire skin, concentrating on the drier areas. Then blot off any excess from the oily areas with a tissue.

Right: A twin approach to skincare will double the benefits for combination skin, and it needn't be time consuming.

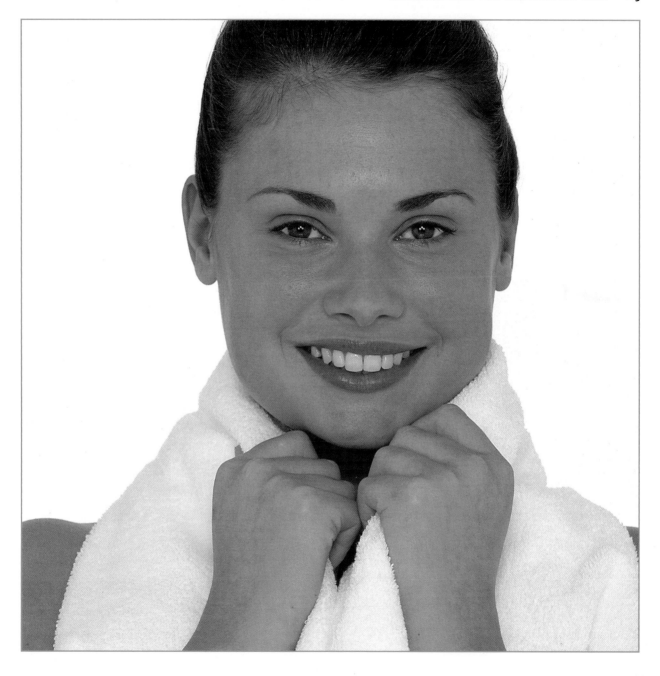

Soothing Care for Sensitive Skin

Sensitive skin is usually quite fine in texture, with a tendency to be rosier than usual. Easily irritated by products and external factors, it's also prone to redness and allergy and may have fine broken veins across the cheeks and nose. There are varying levels of sensitivity. If you feel you can't use any products on your skin without irritating it, cleanse with whole milk and moisturize with a solution of glycerin and rosewater. These should soothe it.

CARING FOR SENSITIVE SKIN

Your skin needs extra-gentle products to keep it healthy. Choose from hypoallergenic ranges that are specially formulated to protect sensitive skin. They're screened for common irritants, such as fragrance, that can cause dryness, itchiness or even an allergic reaction. Remember to moisturize your skin well as dryness can make sensitive skin even more uncomfortable. Don't forget to choose an unperfumed moisturizer.

Tip
If you have particularly sensitive skin, try using an evening primrose oil moisturizer. It's a wonderful natural moisturizer, particularly for dry or very dry skins, as it hydrates, protects and soothes. It also improves the skin's overall softness and suppleness. Many sufferers of eczema also find it useful.

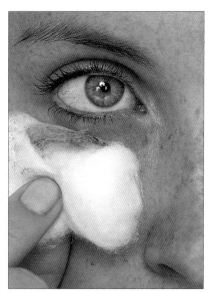

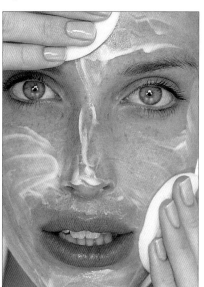

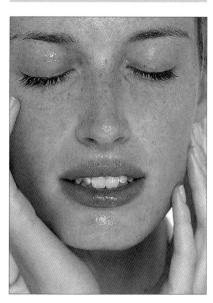

1 Make sure that the make-up you use is hypoallergenic, too, and remove it thoroughly. First use a soothing eye make-up remover. Apply with a cotton wool (cotton ball) pad, then remove every last trace with a clean cotton bud (swab).

2 Avoid facial washes and soaps on your skin, as these are likely to strip the skin of oil and moisture, which can increase your skin's sensitivity even more. So, instead, choose a light, hypoallergenic cleansing lotion.

3 Even the mildest skin freshener can break down the natural protection your delicate skin needs against the elements. So freshen it by simply splashing with warm water instead. This will also remove the final traces of cleanser and eye make-up remover from your skin.

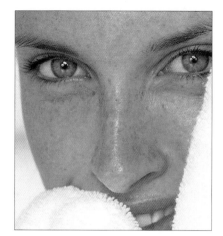

4 Lightly pat your face dry with a soft towel, taking care not to rub the skin as this could irritate it.

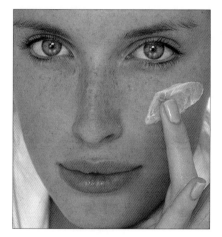

5 It's essential to keep your skin well moisturized to strengthen it and provide a barrier against irritants that can lead to sensitivity.

Right: Careful skincare will take the sting out of sensitive skins.

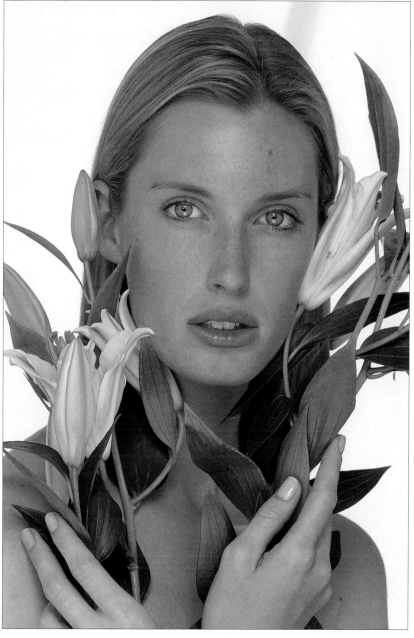

Try a Fabulous Facial

For deep-down cleansing and a definite improvement in skin tone, try an at-home facial. Just once a month will make a noticeable difference to your complexion. Follow these steps to re-create the benefits of the beauty salon in the comfort and privacy of your own home.

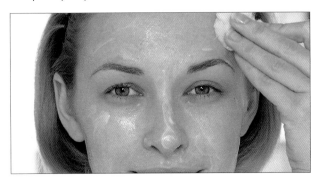

1 Smooth your skin with cleansing cream. Leave on for 1-2 minutes to give it time to dissolve grime, oils and stale make-up. Then gently smooth away excess cream with cotton wool pads (cotton balls).

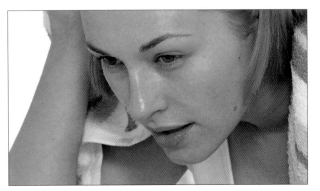

2 Dampen your skin with warm water, then gently massage in a blob of facial scrub using your fingertips, avoiding the delicate eye area. This will loosen dead surface skin cells and leave your skin softer and smoother. It will also prepare your complexion for the beneficial treatments to come. Rinse with warm water.

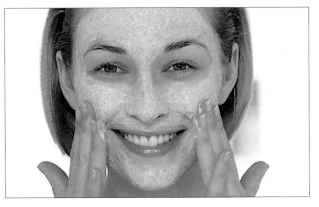

3 Fill a wash basin (sink) with boiling water. Lean over the top, capturing the steam with a towel draped over your head. Stay there for five minutes and then gently remove any blackheads with tissue-covered fingers. If you have sensitive skin, or broken veins, you should avoid this step.

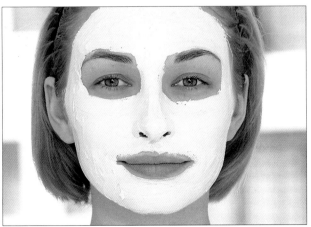

4 Smooth on a face mask. Choose a clay-based one if you have oily skin, or a moisturizing one if you have dry or normal skin. Leave on for five minutes, or for as long as specified by the instructions on the product.

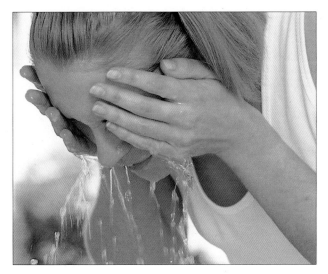

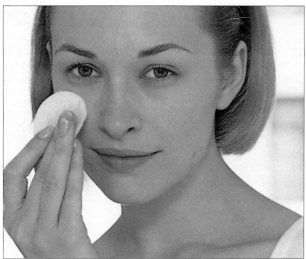

5 Rinse away the face mask with warm water. Finish off with a few splashes of cool water to close your pores and freshen your skin, then pat dry with a towel.

6 Soak a cotton wool (cotton ball) pad with a skin toner lotion and smooth over oily areas, such as the T-zone on the nose, chin and forehead.

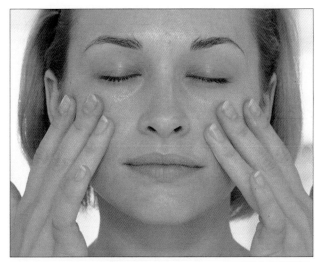

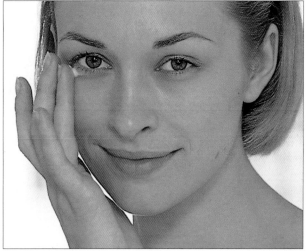

7 Dot your skin with moisturizer and smooth it in. Take the opportunity to massage your skin, as this encourages a brighter complexion and can help reduce puffiness.

8 Smooth the sensitive eye area under your eyes with a soothing eye cream to reduce fine lines and wrinkles, and make the skin ultrasoft.

Delicate Care for Eyes

The fine skin around the eyes is the first to show the signs of ageing, as well as dark circles and puffiness. It needs extra special care because it's thinner than the skin on the rest of your face, so it's less able to hold in moisture. There are also fewer oil glands in this area, which adds to the potential dryness, and there's no fatty layer underneath the skin to act as a shock absorber. The result is that this skin quickly loses it elasticity.

CHOOSING AN EYE TREATMENT

Face creams and oils are too heavy for the eye area. They can block tear ducts, causing puffiness, so you should choose a specific eye treatment that won't aggravate your skin. There are hundreds of products to choose from. Gel-based ones are great for young or oily skins and are refreshing to use. However, most women find light eye creams and balms are gentler and more suitable.

Apply a tiny amount of the eye treatment with your ring finger, as this is the weakest one on your hand. It's better to apply it regularly in small quantities than to apply lots only occasionally. This will help keep your skin more supple and prevent premature wrinkling in this area.

Right: Try placing cucumber slices over the eyelids – they are a natural aid for puffy eyes.

Far right: Cotton wool pads (cotton balls) soaked in rosewater and put over the eyelids soothe tired eyes.

DE-PUFFING EYES

This is one of the most common beauty problems. These ideas can help:

■ Gently tap your skin with your ring finger when you're applying eye cream to encourage the excess fluid to drain away.

■ Store creams in the refrigerator, as the coldness will also help reduce puffiness.

■ Take a couple of slices of cucumber (or strips of grated potato) and rest them on your eyes for 20 minutes.

■ Rest for about 15 minutes with two damp tea bags over your eyes; tea bags are said to help fade under-eye bags because they contain tannin and polyphenols which have an astringent effect.

■ Fill a small bowl with iced water or ice-cold milk. Soak a cotton wool (cotton ball) pad with the liquid and lie down with the dampened pads over your eyes. Replace the pads as soon as they become warm. Continue for 15 minutes. As well as reducing puffiness, this treatment will brighten the whites of your eyes.

■ Soak two cotton wool wedges (cotton balls) in chilled rosewater, squeeze out the excess and rest them on your eyes for 20 minutes.

■ Leave a teaspoon in the fridge for an hour or overnight, remove it and place the bulb of the spoon over your eye, first making sure it is not too cold or freezing, as this may damage your skin.

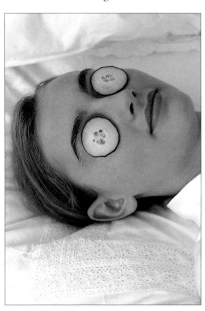

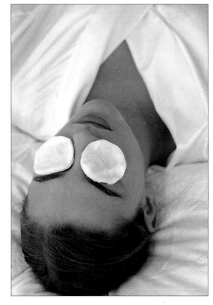

Good Night Creams

Going to bed with night cream on your face can benefit your skin while you sleep. Your skin's cell renewal is more active during the night, and night creams are designed to make the most of these hours. Using a night cream gives your skin the chance to repair the daily wear and tear caused by pollution, make-up and ultraviolet light.

What are night creams?

The main difference between night creams and ordinary daily moisturizers is that most night creams have added ingredients such as vitamins and anti-ageing components. They can be thicker and more intensive than day creams because you don't need to wear make-up on top of them.

Who needs night creams?

While very young skins don't really need the extra nourishing properties of night creams, most women find that they benefit from using one. Dry and very dry skins respond particularly well. You don't have to choose very rich formulations, as there are now lighter alternatives that contain the same special ingredients. Choose the best formulation on the basis of how dry your skin is – it shouldn't feel overloaded.

> **Tip**
> Applying night cream to slightly damp skin can really boost its performance, as this helps to seal in extra moisture – which means softer and smoother skin the next morning.

Below left: Applying night cream just before you go to bed means waking up to a softer complexion.

Below: Dry areas, like cheeks, will absorb the extra moisture a rich night cream can provide.

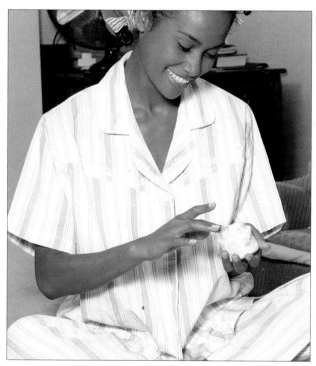

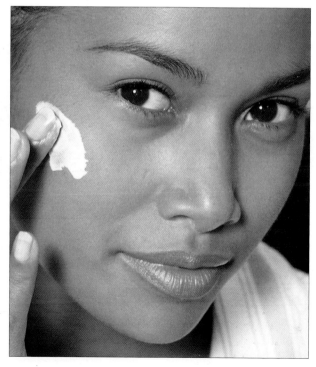

Miraculous Masks

If there's one skincare item that can work immediate miracles, it's a face mask. But, like any other skincare product, you can't just reach for the first one and hope for the best. You should choose carefully to pick the perfect product for you.

MASK IT!

Choose from the wonderful selection of face masks on the market.

Moisturizing masks

Suitable for dry complexions, these rich masks will boost the moisture levels of your skin. This means they can help banish dry patches, flakiness and even fine lines. They work quickly like an intensive moisturizer and are usually left on the skin for 5-10 minutes before being removed with tissue. The slight residue left on the skin will continue to work until it is next cleansed. They're a great treat, particularly after sunbathing, or when your skin feels "tight".

Clay and mud masks

Oily skins need a clay or mud mask to absorb excess grease and impurities from the skin. They're an ideal way to "shrink" open pores, blot out shininess and clear away troublesome blemishes. They dry on your skin over a period of 5-15 minutes, then you simply wash them away with warm water, rinsing dead skin cells, dirt and grime away at the same time. They're a great pick-me-up for skin.

Exfoliating masks

These deep-cleansing masks keep your skin in tip-top condition. Even normal skins sometimes suffer from the build-up of dead skin cells, which can create a dull look and lead to future problems, such as blackheads. Masks that cleanse and exfoliate are the perfect solution. They smooth on like a clay mask and are left to dry. When you rinse them away, their tiny abrasive particles wash away the skin's surface debris.

Peel-off masks

Try this technique; it's great for all skin types and fun to use. You smooth on the gel, leave it to dry, then peel it away. The light formulation will help refresh oily areas by clearing clogged pores, as well as lightly nourishing drier skins.

Gel masks

Gel masks are suitable for sensitive skins, as well as oily complexions, as they have a wonderfully soothing and cooling effect. You simply apply the gel, lie back and relax, then after 5-10 minutes remove the excess with tissue. They're wonderful after too much sun, or when your skin feels irritated.

Below: Clay and mud masks dry on your skin over a period of 5-15 minutes.

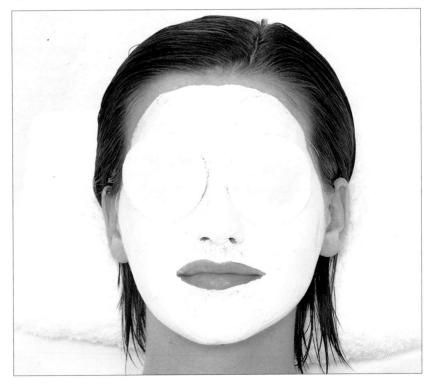

Facial Scrubs

Brighten up your complexion in an instant with this skincare treat. If you don't include a facial scrub in your weekly skincare regime, then you've been missing out. Technically known as exfoliation, it's a simple method that removes dead surface cells from the top of your skin, revealing the plumper, younger ones underneath. It also encourages your skin to speed up cell production, which means that the cells that reach the surface are younger and better looking. The result is a brighter, smoother complexion – no matter what your age.

ACTION TACTICS

Use an exfoliator on dry or normal skin once a week. Oily or combination skins can be exfoliated once or twice a week. As a rule, avoid this treatment on sensitive skin, or if you have bad acne. However, you can gently exfoliate pimple-prone skin once a week to help keep pores clear and to prevent breakouts.

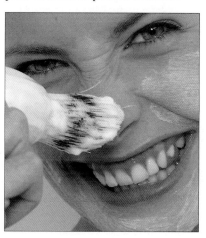

GETTING TO THE NITTY-GRITTY

■ Apply a blob of facial scrub cream to damp skin, massage gently, then rinse away with lots of cool water. Opt for an exfoliator that contains gentler, rounded beads, rather than scratchy ones like crushed kernels.

■ Try a mini exfoliating pad, lathering up with soap or facial wash.

Tip

Whichever method of exfoliation you choose to use, avoid scrubbing the delicate area around the eyes. This is because the skin is very fine here and it can easily be irritated.

Below: Get your skin glowing with a quick and easy facial treat.

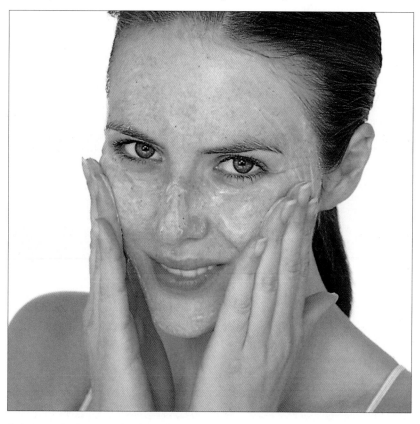

Left: Instead of using a facial scrub, gently massage your skin with a soft flannel (wash cloth), facial brush, or old, clean shaving brush.

Be a Fruity Beauty

Incorporated in small amounts, alpha-hydroxy acids (AHAs) have recently become a key ingredient in specialized skincare products. They've become the biggest skincare invention of the 1990s, and their success looks set to continue for many years. Many women find AHAs dramatically improve the condition and look of their skin.

AHA KNOW-HOW

Alpha-hydroxy acids, also commonly known as fruit acids, are found in natural products. These include citric acid from citrus fruit, lactic acid from sour milk, tartaric acid from wine, and malic acid from apples and other fruits.

AHAs work by breaking down the protein bonds that hold together the dead cells on the surface of your skin. They then lift them away and reveal the brighter, plumper cells underneath. This gentle process cleans and clears blocked pores, improves your skin tone and softens the look of fine lines. You should start to see results within a couple of weeks, although many women report that they see an improvement after only a few days.

Without even realizing the exact reasons for their improved skin, women have used AHAs for centuries. For example, Cleopatra is said to have bathed in sour asses' milk, and ladies of the French court applied wine to their faces to keep their skin smooth, supple and blemish free – both these ancient beauty aids are now known to contain AHAs.

AHA products are best used under your ordinary everyday moisturizer as a treatment cream. You should avoid applying them to the delicate eye and lip areas. If you have very sensitive skin, you may find they're not suitable for you, but some women experience a slight tingling sensation at first anyway, as the product gets to work.

The great news is that AHA products are now becoming more affordable, and not just the preserve of more expensive skincare companies. Many mid-market companies are including the benefits of AHAs in their products, so everyone can give their skin the high-tech treatment it deserves. You can also find AHA products for the hands and body, so you can reap the benefits from head to toe.

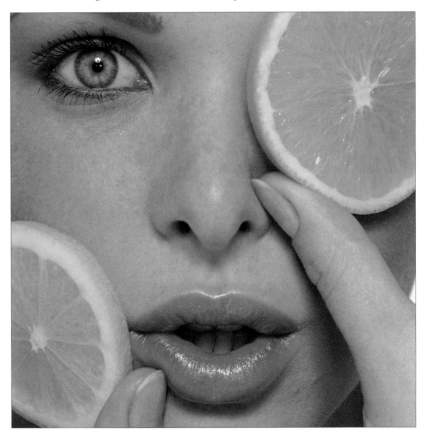

Above: AHAs (otherwise known as fruit acids) are an effective way to put the zing back into your skin. In fact, there's nothing new about AHAs – by bathing in asses' milk Cleopatra was absorbing AHAs into her skin.

Special Skin Treatments

You'd be forgiven for thinking you might need a PhD in chemistry to choose a skin treatment these days! As well as basic moisturizers, there are a whole host of special treatments, serums and gels that are designed to treat specific problems.

THE KEY TREATMENTS

You'll find that special skin treatments come in all shapes and sizes and in various formulations.

Serums and gels

These products have an ultra-light formulation, a non-greasy texture and a high concentration of active ingredients. They're not usually designed to be used on their own, except on oily skins. They're generally applied under a moisturizer to enhance its benefits and boost the anti-ageing process.

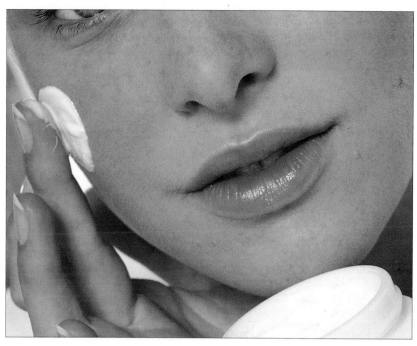

Above: Choose a cream that contains specialized ingredients to improve your skin.

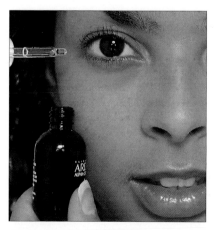

Above: Try using a few drops of special skin serum — it will work wonders for your skin.

Skin firmers

These creams are designed to tighten, firm and smooth your skin. They work by forming an ultra-fine film on the skin, which tightens your complexion and reduces the appearance of fine lines. The effects last for a few hours, and make-up can easily be applied on top. These products are a wonderful treat for a special night out or when you're feeling particularly tired.

Skin energizers

Speed up the natural production and repair of your skin cells with these creams that contain special ingredients. As well as producing a fresher, younger-looking skin, skin energizers are also thought to help combat the signs of ageing.

Ampule treatments

These special treatments are very concentrated active ingredients contained in sealed glass phials or ampules, to ensure that they're completely fresh. Typical extracts include herbs, wheat germ, vitamins and collagen – used for their intensive and fast-acting results. Vitamin E is another great, natural skin saver and healer. Break open a capsule and smooth the oil onto your face for an immediate skin treat.

10 Ways to Beat Wrinkles

Fine lines and wrinkles aren't inevitable. In fact, skin experts believe that most skin damage can be prevented with a little know-how and some special care. Here are the 10 main points to bear in mind, no matter what your age.

1 Protect your skin from the sun

The single biggest cause of skin ageing is sunlight. You should use a sunscreen every single day of the year. This will help prevent your skin from becoming prematurely aged, as well as guard against burning and of course the risk of skin cancer. The ageing rays of the sun are as prevalent in the cold winter months as in the hot summer ones, so it's a daily safeguard you should take.

2 Stop smoking

Cigarette smoke speeds up the ageing process because it strips your skin of oxygen and slows down the rate at which new cells are regenerated. It's responsible for giving the skin a grey, sluggish look, and it can also cause fine lines around the mouth because heavy smokers tend to be constantly pursing their lips to draw on a cigarette.

3 Deep cleanse

It's essential to ensure that your skin is clear of dead skin cells, dirt and make-up to give it a youthful, fresh glow. You don't have to use harsh products to do this – a creamy cleanser removed with cotton wool (cotton balls) is a good option for most women. If your skin is very dry, try massaging it with an oily cleanser. Leave it on your skin for a few minutes, then rinse away the excess with warm water.

4 Deep moisturize

You can either use a nourishing face mask, or apply a thick layer of your usual moisturizer or night cream to boost the water levels of your skin on a weekly basis. Whichever you choose, leave it on the skin for 5-10 minutes, then remove the excess with tissues. Apply to damp skin for greater effect.

5 Boost the circulation

Buy a gentle facial scrub or exfoliator, and use once a week to keep the surface of your skin soft and smooth. This will

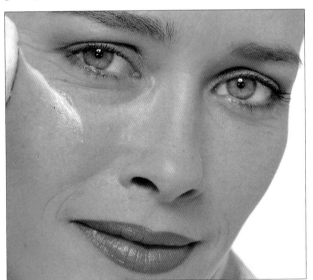

Above: You won't believe the difference regular cleansing can make to your skin.

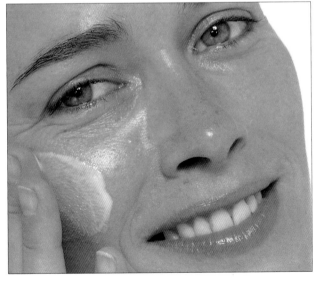

Above: Protect and survive by using a good moisturizer on a regular basis.

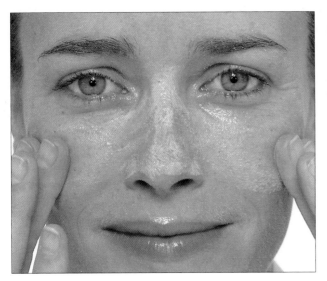

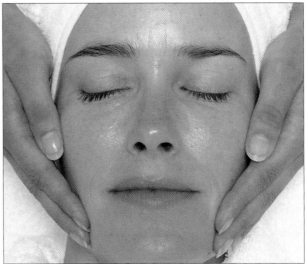

also increase the blood flow to the top layers of the skin, giving it a rosy glow and helping to encourage cell renewal. Alternatively, you can get the same effect by lathering up a facial wash on your skin using a clean shaving brush.

6 Disguise lines

Existing lines can be minimized to the naked eye by opting for the latest light-reflecting foundations, concealers and powders. These contain luminescent particles that bounce light away from your skin, making lines less noticeable and giving your skin a wonderful fresh-faced luminosity.

7 Pamper regularly

As well as a regular skincare regime, remember to treat your skin occasionally to special treatments such as facials, serums and anti-ageing creams. As well as improving the look of your skin, they'll encourage you to give it extra care on a regular basis.

8 Be weather vain

Extremes of cold and hot weather can strip your skin of essential moisture, leaving it dry and more prone to damage. Central heating can have the same effect. For this reason, ensure that you moisturize regularly, changing your products according to the seasons.

For instance, you may need a more oily product in the winter that will keep the cold out and won't freeze on the skin's surface. In hot weather, lighter formulations are more comfortable on the skin, and you can boost their activity by using a few drops of special treatment serum underneath.

9 Be gentle

Be careful you don't drag at your skin when applying skincare products or make-up. The skin around your eyes is particularly vulnerable. So, make sure you always use a light touch, and whenever you can, use upward and outward strokes, rather than dragging the

Above left: Wake up to the benefits of special skincare treatments.
Above: Relax and enjoy a beneficial facial - you'll reap the rewards.

skin down. When applying under-eye skin products, tap the cream on gently with the tip of your ring finger. Also, be careful to avoid any products that make your skin itch, sting or feel sensitive. If any product causes this sort of reaction, stop using it at once, and switch to a gentler formulation.

10 Clever make-up

Skincare benefits aren't just confined to skincare products these days. so investigate some of the latest make-up on offer. In fact, many make-up products now contain ultraviolet (UV) filters and skin-nourishing ingredients to treat your skin as well as superficially improve its appearance. So investigate the latest products – it's well worth making use of them for 24-hour-a-day benefits.

How Well do you Care for your Body?

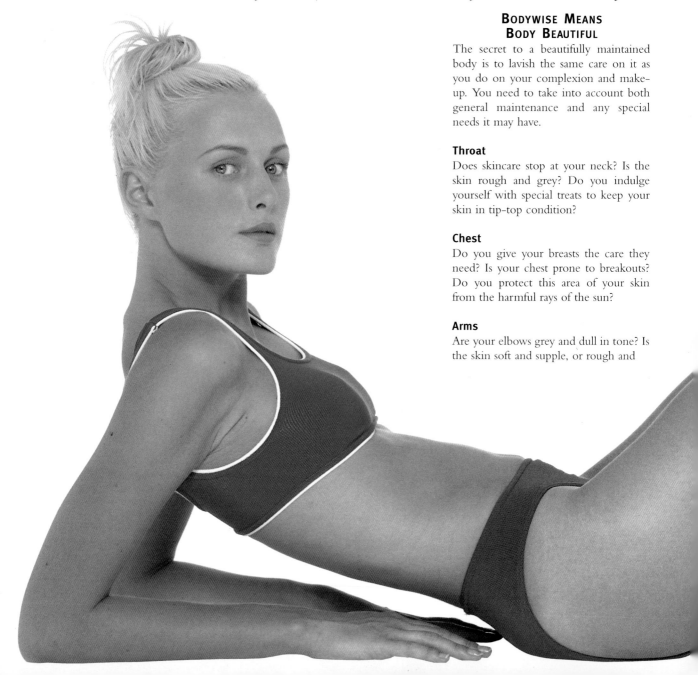

The secret to a beautifully maintained body is to lavish the same care on it as you do on your complexion and make-up. You need to take into account both general maintenance and any special needs it may have.

Throat

Does skincare stop at your neck? Is the skin rough and grey? Do you indulge yourself with special treats to keep your skin in tip-top condition?

Chest

Do you give your breasts the care they need? Is your chest prone to breakouts? Do you protect this area of your skin from the harmful rays of the sun?

Arms

Are your elbows grey and dull in tone? Is the skin soft and supple, or rough and dry? Do darker hairs on your lower arms need bleaching? If you remove hair from your underarms, have you found the best method, the one that suits you for both convenience and results? Have you found the solution to underarm freshness?

Hands

Do your hands need moisturizing care? Are your nails neatly filed and shaped? Would a lick of polish or a French manicure give them a helping hand? Do you need to stop biting your nails?

Legs

Are your legs free from stubbly hair? Is the skin as smooth as it could be? Would they benefit from a light touch of fake tan? Are they prone to cellulite? Would bath time treats improve the look and feel of your skin?

Bikini line

If you remove hair from this area, have you found the best method for you?

Feet

Are your feet free from hard skin, corns and calluses? Are your nails neatly trimmed? Do you smooth a foot cream on them regularly to ensure that the skin stays soft?

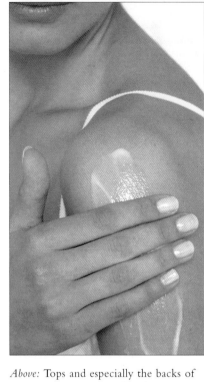

Above: Tops and especially the backs of arms need care too, so that they stay soft, supple and firm.

Bathroom Essentials

Caring for your body creates endless rewards. So, keep a selection of beauty products on hand to maintain your skin from head to toe on a daily and occasional basis.

BATHING BEAUTY

The time of day and even the time of year will affect what you like using, so why not take the opportunity to try different products, adding the ones you particularly like to those you already know well and use frequently.

Soaps and cleansing bars

These are a cheap and effective way of cleansing your body. If you find them too drying, choose ones that contain moisturizers to minimize these effects. Most people can use ordinary soaps and cleansers without any problem. However, if you have particularly dry or sensitive skin, opt for the pH-balanced variety.

Shower gels and bubble baths

Gels and bubbles provide mild detergents that cleanse your body while you soak in the water. There are hundreds of varieties to choose from, including those containing a host of additives, ranging from herbs to essential oils. If you find them too harsh for your skin, look for the ones that offer 2-in-1 benefits – these contain moisturizers as well, to soothe your skin.

Sponges and washcloths

Dislodge dirt and grime with a sponge or washcloth. They are also useful for lathering up soaps and gels on your skin. Wash your washcloth regularly, and allow it to dry between uses. Natural sponges are a more expensive but long-lasting alternative. Squeeze out afterwards in warm clear water and allow to dry naturally. However, don't underestimate the power of your hands for washing yourself; they keep you in touch with your body and will make you aware of any lumps, bumps and changes in texture that might occur.

Below: Wonder bars for the body.

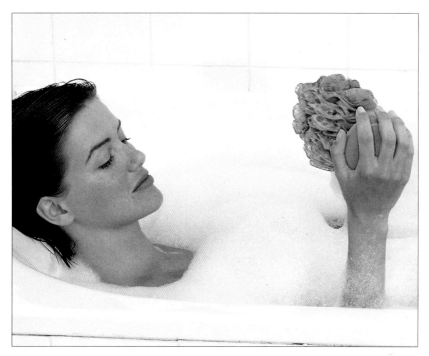

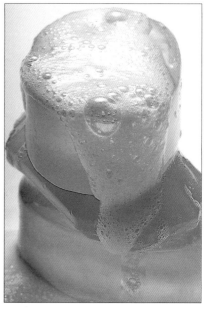

Left: Bubbles, bubbles – soothe away toils and troubles!

Bath oils

Oils for the bath are a wonderful beauty boon for those with dry skins. They float on the top of the water, and your entire body becomes covered with a fine film when you step out of the bath. Most cosmetic houses produce a bath oil, but if you're not worried about the fragrance, you can use a few drops of any vegetable oil, such as olive, corn or peanut.

Bath salts

Special salts made from sodium carbonate are particularly useful for softening hard water and for preventing your skin from becoming too dry. Combined with warm water, they're a popular way to soothe away aches and pains.

Below: Stock your bathroom shelves for head-to-toe freshness.

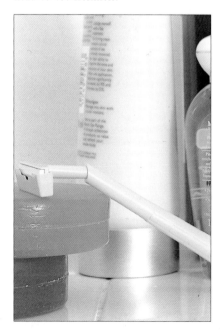

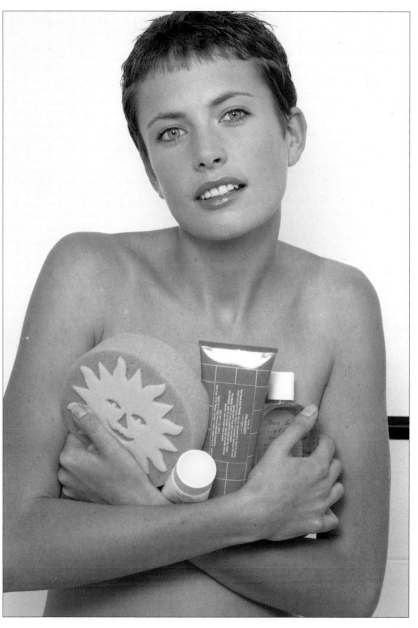

Above: Grab yourself some bathroom benefits.

Bathroom Treatments

As well as a chance to cleanse your body, bath or shower time is the perfect opportunity to pamper and polish your skin, and indulge in some beauty treats. Try some of these effective body treats on a regular basis.

Body lotions and oils

Seal moisture into your skin with a lotion or oil, making it soft and smooth. Especially concentrate on drier areas, such as feet, elbows and knees. Oilier and normal skins benefit from lotions, while oils and creams suit drier skins.

Exfoliating scrubs

Help combat the rough patches and blackheads that can appear on your skin by using a scrub. Use once or twice a week in the bath or shower, rinsing away the excess with clear warm water.

Pumice stone

These stones, made from very porous volcanic rock, work best if you lather up with soap before rubbing at hardened areas of skin in a circular motion. Don't rub too fiercely or else you'll make the skin sore. A little and often is best.

Loofahs and back brushes

Back brushes or long loofahs are useful as exfoliators, and their length makes them great for scrubbing difficult-to-reach areas like the back. Loofahs are actually the pod of an Egyptian plant and need a bit of care if they're to last. Rinse and drain them thoroughly after use to stop them going black and mouldy. Avoid rinsing them in vinegar and lemon juice as this can be too harsh for these once-living things. Back brushes are easier to care for; you simply rinse them in cool water after use and leave them to dry.

BATH TIME TREATS

Soaking in a warm bath has to be one of the most popular ways to relax. You can literally feel your cares disappear as you sink into the soothing water. However, you can also use bath time for a variety of other benefits and beauty boosters.

Learning to relax

Turn bathtime into an aromatherapy treat by adding relaxing essential oils such as chamomile and lavender to the water. Just add a few drops once you've run the bath, then lie back, inhale the vapours and relax. Salts and bubble baths that contain sea minerals and kelp also have a relaxing effect and purify your skin, too. Bathe by candlelight and listen to soothing music to make it even more of a treat. Put on eye pads and relax for 10 minutes.

BE A NATURAL BEAUTY

You don't have to splash out on expensive bath additives – try making your own:

■ Soothe irritated skin by adding a cup of cider vinegar to the running water.

■ A cup of powdered milk will soothe rough skin.

■ Add a cupful of oatmeal or bran to cleanse, whiten and soothe your skin.

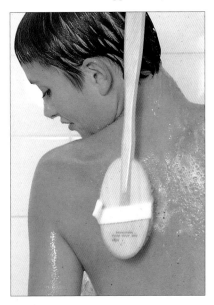

Above: Get back to basics with a brush to reach difficult areas.

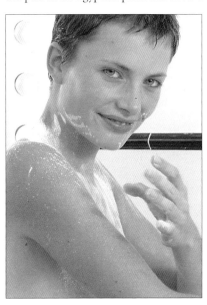

Above: Powder power for fresh, dry skin.

Sleek skin

Smooth your body with body oil before getting into the bath. After soaking for 10 minutes, rub your skin with a soft washcloth – you'll be amazed at how much dead skin you remove.

Boosting benefits

If you pat yourself dry after a bath, it'll help you to unwind, whereas briskly rubbing your skin with a towel will help to invigorate you.

SHOWER TIME TREATS

Showers are a wonderful opportunity to cleanse your body quickly, cheaply and to wake yourself up. Here are some of the other benefits.

Circulation booster

Switch on the cold water before finishing your shower to help boost your circulation. Strangely, it will also make you feel warmer once you get out of the shower. It also works well if you concentrate the blasts of cold water on cellulite-prone areas, as this stimulates the sluggish circulation in these spots.

Right: Splish! Splash! Relax and have fun in the bath.

Below: Turn a daily shower into a real power shower.

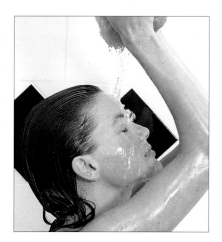

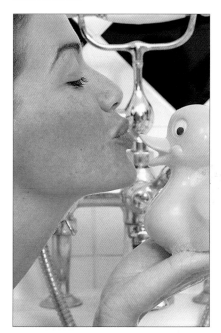

Above: Bath time is more fun if you share it.

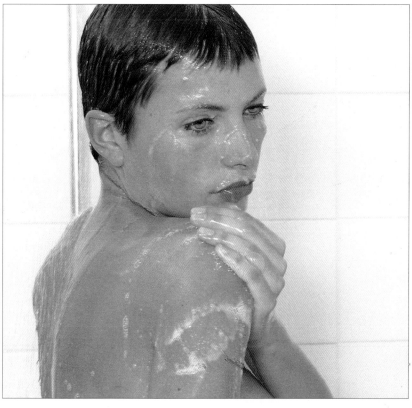

Your Bodycare Routine

When your mind is fixed on fast improvement, it is important to think about taking care of your whole body. For example, rough, mottled skin detracts from an otherwise great figure, but if it's smooth it will improve a not-so-perfect figure – and make a good one look even better.

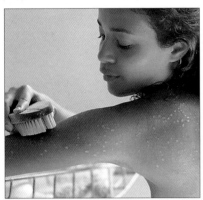

1 Body brushes can be used in the water. Do not use so vigorously that you damage the skin.

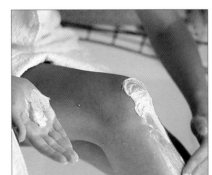

2 Remember to exfoliate the skin on your legs for all-over smoothness.

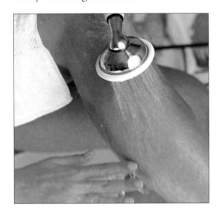

3 After exfoliating, spritz the skin with intermittent bursts of warm and then cool water to boost circulation and skin tone.

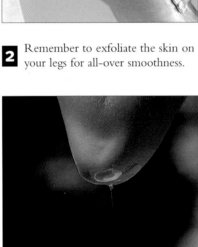

4 After spritzing, moisturize your skin. Oil is particularly nourishing for dry skin.

YOUR BASIC ROUTINE

Include the following steps in your bathroom routine and your skin will probably improve dramatically within a few weeks.

Body brush

Brushing your skin – from feet to hips and hands to shoulders – with a natural bristle brush exfoliates and tones. Go gently at first as you might find that your skin feels a bit tender to begin with. However, if you continue using a body brush each day you should be able to build up pressure and your skin will feel less sensitive over time. After body brushing these areas, take a little time to soak in a warm, oily bath to wind down and relax.

Exfoliation

Body exfoliators have larger grains than facial ones because body skin is tougher. It is easiest to buff in a shower or sauna. Try it – once a week or whenever you have time – on areas that are prone to dry skin, such as your elbows, shins, heels, knees, and your hands.

Moisturizing

Pay special attention to thirsty shins, elbows, upper arms, hips and knees; moisturize when your body is slightly damp and warm as creams will sink into the skin much more quickly.

Right: Dry areas such as shins and knees need lots of care, especially during the winter when cold weather removes natural moisture from the skin.

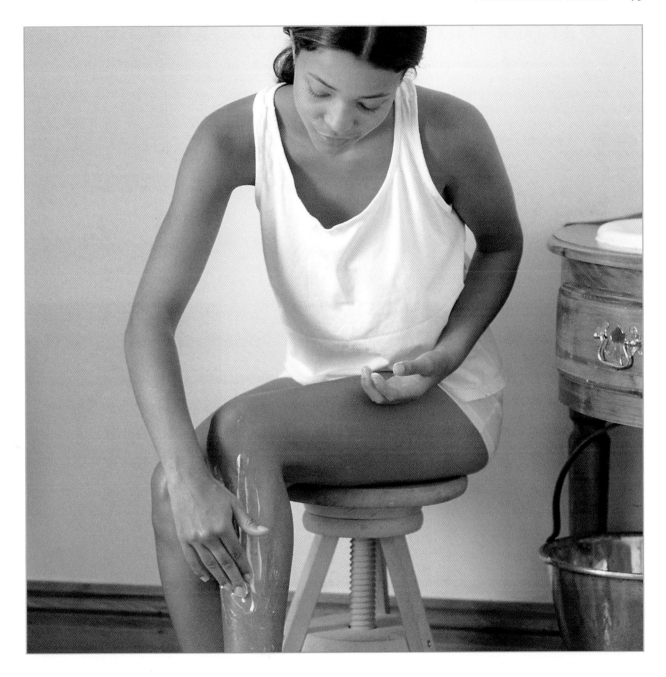

Caring for your Hands and Feet

Most of us do not give our hands and feet the attention they deserve. Our hands are constantly exposed to the elements, to harsh detergents, soaps and hot washing-up water. When our feet hit the ground they absorb nearly five times our body weight — it is important to remember to look after them.

CARING FOR YOUR HANDS

Hands are always visible, so the ideal is to have smooth skin and nicely manicured nails. But our hands are always exposed to the elements. This exposure causes the skin on the backs of our hands to age quickly; liver spots – pigmentation marks that look like oversized freckles – can appear, but these can be lightened with fading creams. To keep the skin on your hands supple, have a bottle of hand lotion by the kitchen sink and, if you dislike wearing rubber gloves, smother your hands with it before putting them into washing-up water or doing any other kind of housework.

Super-supple skin boosters

Manicurists treat hands that are dry to the point of cracking and callousing with skin-softening warm paraffin wax – the skin is coated with it and then peeled off when set. You can renourish really dry hands at home by soaking them in warm olive oil. Fill a teacup with the warmed oil, dip in your fingers and let them soak for a few minutes. When you remove them, rub the oil into your hands.

> **Lemon clean**
> Bleach stained hands naturally using fresh lemon juice; wash them afterwards with mild, unscented soap, and use a pumice stone to remove rough skin; then rub in lots of rich hand cream.

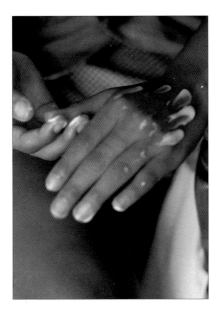

Above: Gently massage hand cream into your hands, remembering to rub it into the skin around the nails. Remove excess with a tissue.

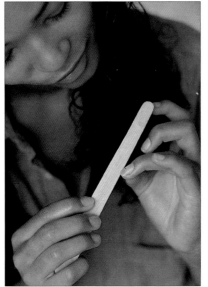

Above: Fingernails should be filed regularly. To minimize breakage, file them straight across with a soft emery board.

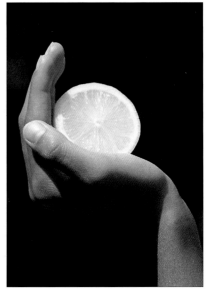

Above: The juice of a lemon is a good natural bleach for both hands and nails.

CARING FOR YOUR FEET

If you take care of your feet – keeping toenails trimmed, removing rough skin, and massaging feet and ankles regularly – you should not have any problems. This simple footcare routine does not take long – enjoy it a couple of times a week.

■ Remove any hard skin with a pumice stone or sloughing cream. If you use a foot file, rub your skin very gently before rinsing off the flaky residue.

■ Dry your feet well, especially between your toes; trim your toenails by cutting straight across the tip (but not down the sides), and file sharp corners with an emery board.

■ Soak your feet for a minimum of five minutes in a bowl or tub of hot water to which you have added some mineral salts or plain sea salt. Bubble foot spas are a good treat for feet; add a couple of drops of lavender essential oil to soothe aches and ease swelling.

■ Massage your feet by cupping your hands on either side of your foot and, using your thumbs, firmly pressing the upper part of your foot while pushing your thumbs down and outwards to the sides of your foot. Grasp each ankle and gently massage the ankle bone in circular movements to ease any stiffness. Work each foot in turn.

■ If your feet are feeling tired or swollen, try resting your feet above your head for 10 minutes. Do this by lying at right angles to a wall, or on the floor with your feet resting on the edge of a chair. Any swelling will disappear as trapped fluids travel back up your legs towards your heart.

Corn cures
Never try to tackle a corn yourself with a foot file, but go to a chiropodist. Soaking your feet in warm, soapy water will help to soften corns, and padded rings – which you can buy from a pharmacist – will ease the pressure.

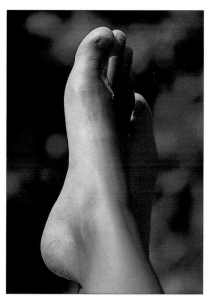

Above: After a long winter it may come as a shock to reveal your feet; it's important to keep the skin on your feet nourished and smooth.

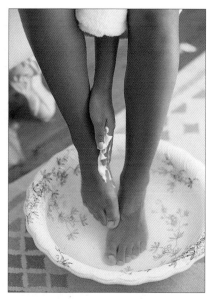

Above: To soften and remove dry skin, first soak your feet in warm water and cleanse thoroughly. Then use a foot file or pumice stone to remove the dry skin.

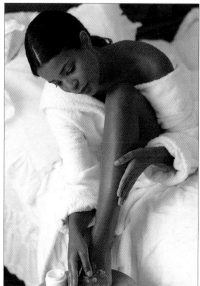

Above: After you have gently filed your feet with a foot file, smooth on foot cream to nourish and further soften the skin on your feet.

Scrub your Way to Smoother Skin

Improve your skin tone from head to toe with the regular use of a body scrub. This quick treatment is easy to do and boasts great results. The chances are, even if your skin isn't prone to spottiness or flaky patches, it will suffer from dullness and poor condition from time to time. This is where body scrubs and exfoliators come into their own. They work by shifting dead cells from the surface of your skin, revealing the younger, fresher ones underneath. This process also stimulates the circulation of blood in the skin tissues, giving it a rosy glow.

METHODS TO TRY

There are lots of different ways you can exfoliate your body – so there's one to suit every budget and preference.

■ An exfoliating scrub is a cream- or gel-based product containing tiny abrasive particles. Use the type with rounded particles, which won't scratch and irritate delicate skin. Simply massage the scrub into damp skin, then rinse away thoroughly with lots of warm water.

■ A bath mitt, loofah or sisal mitt are a cinch to use and cost effective, too. They can be quite harsh on the skin if you press too hard, so go easy at first. Simply sweep over your body when you're in the shower or bath. Rinse them well after use, and allow them to dry naturally.

■ Your ordinary washcloth or bath sponge can also double up as an exfoliator. Lather up with plenty of soap or shower gel, and massage over damp skin before rinsing away with clear water.

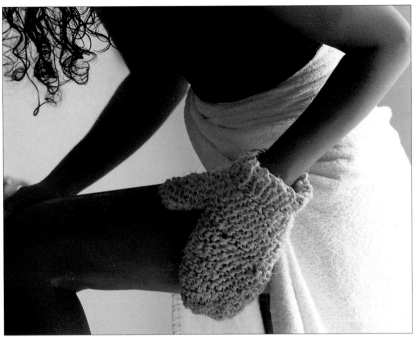

Above: Keep a sisal mitt to hand for super soft skin.

■ Copy what health spas do, and keep a large tub of natural sea salt by the shower. Scoop up a handful when you get in, and massage over your skin. Rinse away thoroughly afterwards.

■ Make your own body scrub by mixing sea salt with body oil or olive oil. Allow the mixture to soak into your skin for a few minutes to allow the edges of the salt to dissolve before massaging in. Rinse throughly with plenty of water.

■ Body brushes are also useful. The best way to use them is on dry skin before you get in the bath or shower, as this is particularly good for loosening dead skin cells. You can also use them in the water, lathering them up with soap or gel. Try building up pressure gradually over several weeks. Just take care that you don't get too enthusiastic with the brushing and scrub your skin so vigorously that it becomes tender and sore.

Tip
For super-soft skin fast, you should massage your body with oil first before getting into the bath or shower. Then follow the exfoliating method you prefer.

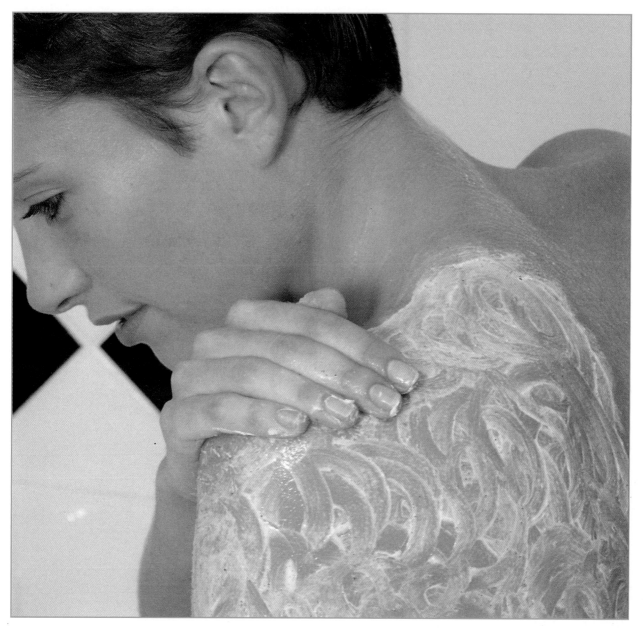

Above: Regular exfoliating works!

Simple Steps to Softer Skin

Slick on a body moisturizer to create a wonderfully silky body. Add a moisturizing body treat every day to your beauty regime, and you will soon reap the benefits.

MOISTURIZING MATTERS

Just as you choose a moisturizer for your face with care, you should opt for the best formulation suited to the skin type on your body.

■ Gels are the lightest formulation and are perfect for very hot days or oilier skin types. They contain a lot of nourishing ingredients even though they're very easy to wear.

■ Lotions and oils are good for most skin types. They are also easy to apply, as they're not too sticky.

■ Creams give better results for those with dry skins, especially very dry areas.

BODY MOISTURIZING

Here are a few tips to help you make the most of moisturizing your body.

■ Apply using firm strokes to boost your circulation as you massage in the product.

■ Apply the moisturizer straight onto clean, damp skin – after a bath or shower is the ideal time. This helps to seal moisture into the upper layers of your skin.

■ Soften cracked feet by rubbing them with rich body lotion, pulling on a pair of cotton socks and heading for bed. They'll be beautifully soft by the next morning!

■ Concentrate on rubbing moisturizer into particularly dry areas, such as heels, knees and elbows. The calves of the legs are also very prone to dryness because there aren't many oil glands there.

■ If you don't have time to apply moisturizer after your bath, simply add a few drops of body oil to the water. When you step out of the bath, your skin will be coated with a fine film of nourishing oil. Remember to rinse the bath well afterwards to prevent you from slipping the next time you take a dip.

■ Your breasts don't have any supportive muscle from the nipple to the collarbone and the skin is very fine here. Using firming creams and body lotions regularly won't work miracles, but they can help maintain the elasticity and suppleness in this delicate area.

Smelling scentsational

Opt for a scented body lotion as a wonderful treat. Applied as a lotion, the scent can be longer lasting than the actual fragrances themselves. Alternatively, use them as part of "fragrance layering". This simply means taking advantage of the various scent formulations that are now available. Start with a scented bath oil and soap, move onto the matching body lotion and powder, and leave the house wearing the fragrance itself sprayed onto pulse points.

However, be careful you don't clash fragrances. Opt for unscented products if you're also wearing a perfume, unless you're going to be wearing a matching scented body lotion. You don't want a whole range of cheaper products competing or clashing with your more expensive perfume.

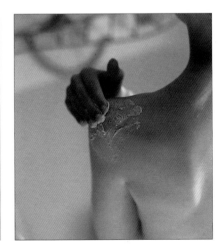

Above: Opt for the light touch with a moisturizing gel.

Above: Shoulders and upper arms benefit from exfoliation before moisturizing.

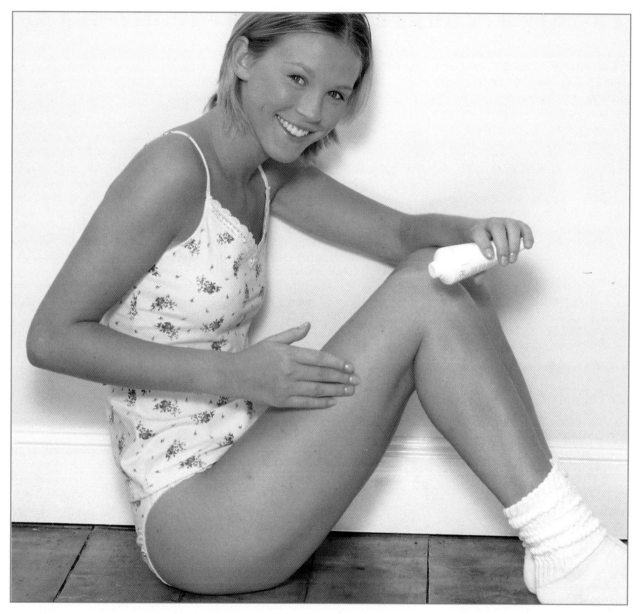

Above: Take the time before dressing to moisturize your skin. Why not apply body lotion and then let your skin absorb it whilst you clean your teeth or dry your hair?

Indulge yourself with Aromatherapy

Aromatherapy is one of the most popular therapies around today. It's wonderful to use, the products are easily available, and they can provide you with immediate results. Aromatherapy uses essential oils, which are distilled essences of herbs, plants, flowers and trees. Most of these oils smell wonderful and are a pleasure to use. It's this smell that usually attracts people to them for treating a variety of physical and mental conditions, from skin infections to stress. There are three main ways to use essential oils.

In the bath

Add 5-10 drops of your chosen oil to your bath, then sink in and relax. Inhaling the wonderful aromas will soothe your mind, and the oils will also have a beneficial effect on your skin and body. Only pour oil into the bath once it's started to run, or the oil will evaporate with the heat of the water and you'll lose the therapeutic properties of the essential oil before you even get in.

For massage

Mix 3-4 drops of essential oil into 10 ml (2 teaspoons) of neutral carrier oil, such as sweet almond oil, and use to massage your body – or ask someone else to massage you. Alternatively, choose one of the many pre-blended oils currently available on the market. Most aromatherapists believe that you're naturally drawn to the oils that will do you most good at that time.

To perfume your room

Fragrance your room and indulge in the beneficial scent. Clay burners are readily available to diffuse oils into the air. Add the oil to some water in the bowl at the top, then light the night candle underneath. Using the water as a carrier for the essential oil will prevent the oil from burning and help to create sweet-smelling steam to permeate your room. Alternatively, place six drops of your chosen oil in a small bowl of water and put it in a warm place, such as on top of a radiator in winter. There are also ring diffusers you can put under light bulbs to very gently heat the oil, or you can add a few drops of oil to the water in a plant sprayer, and use it to spritz the room whenever you like.

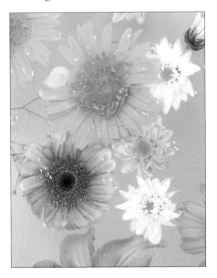

Above: Flower power – treat yourself with fragrant oils from flowers, plants and herbs.

WONDERFUL OILS TO TRY

There are several hundred essential oils to choose from, so it can be confusing knowing which ones to try. These are some useful ones to start with:

Essential oil	Benefits	Use for
Chamomile	calming	headaches and anxiety
Mandarin	calming, refreshing	digestive problems
Eucalyptus	decongestant	colds
Lavender	calming and balancing	stress, colds, headaches, PMT
Peppermint	refreshing	indigestion and sickness
Rose	soothing	depression
Rosemary	antiseptic and stimulating	aches and pains
Sandalwood	relaxing	stress, dry skin care
Tea tree	anti-bacterial	pimples and cold sores
Ylang ylang	love potion	boosting sex drive

Aromatherapy Tips

1 If you don't want to buy individual essential oils buy them ready-blended, or treat yourself to bath and body products that contain them.

2 Some oils are thought to carry some risk during pregnancy. For this reason, consult a qualified aromatherapist for advice if you are expecting a child and want to use essential oils.

3 Don't try to treat medical conditions with them – always consult your doctor.

4 Essential oils can be expensive, but remember that a little goes a long way.

5 Don't apply essential oils to the skin undiluted as they are far too concentrated in this form, and can result in inflammation. The only exception is lavender, which can be used directly on the skin for insect bites and stings. Otherwise essential oils should be mixed with a carrier oil.

6 Don't take essential oils internally. Essential oils are approximately 50-100 times more powerful than the plant they were extracted from.

7 Don't apply oils to areas of broken, inflamed or recently scarred skin.

8 Whichever method of aromatherapy you use, shut the door to the room to prevent the aroma from escaping.

9 For immediate results from aromatherapy, try inhaling the steam. Add about four drops of your chosen oil to a bowl of hot water, lean over it and cover your head with a towel. Inhale deeply for about five minutes.

10 Place a few drops of your favourite oil on a tissue, so you can inhale it whenever you like. Eucalyptus is great if your sinuses are blocked or you have a cold. A few drops of chamomile or lavender on your pillow will help you sleep.

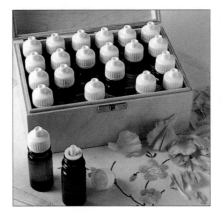

Above: Special essential oils – for a sensual experience.

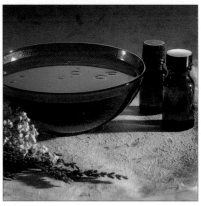

Above: Put a few drops of essential oils into hot water and inhale the steam.

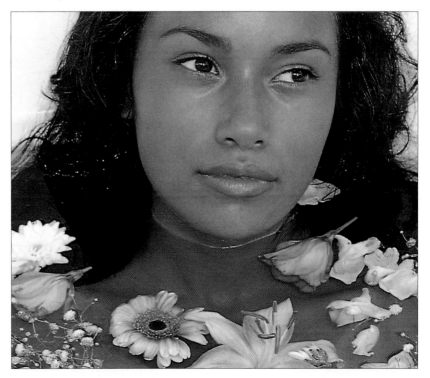

Above: Try a soothing aromatherapy bath, and let your cares float away.

Beat the Cellulite Problem

It's not just plumper, older women who suffer from "orange-peel skin" on their thighs, hips, bottom and even tummy – many slim, young women suffer, too. Despite what you may have heard, there is no miracle cure for cellulite, but there are some effective and practical things you can do to see great results.

FACTS ON CELLULITE

Experts differ about what exactly causes cellulite. It seems likely that it's an accumulation of fat, fluid and toxins trapped into the hardened network of elastin and collagen fibres in the deeper levels of the skin. This causes the dimpled effect and feel of cellulite areas. These areas also tend to feel cold to the touch because the flow of blood is constricted and the lymph system, which is responsible for eliminating toxins, can't work properly. This can worsen the problem and make the cellulite feel puffy and spongy.

HAVE I GOT CELLULITE?

Try squeezing the skin or your upper thigh between your thumb and index finger. If the flesh feels lumpy and looks bumpy, you have cellulite. Further clues may be that these areas look whiter, and feel colder that elsewhere on your legs.

Common causes

Cellulite can be caused and/or aggravated by the following:

■ Hereditary factors – if your mother has cellulite, it's a fair bet you will have, too.

■ Hormones, such as the contraceptive pill, may be contributory.

■ A poor diet is full of toxins and puts the body under great strain to get rid of vast quantities of waste. Also, an unhealthy low-fibre, high-fat diet means that the body's digestive system can't work effectively to expel toxins from the body.

■ Stress and lack of exercise make your body sluggish and can slow down blood circulation and the lymphatic system.

TAKING THE SENSIBLE APPROACH

There are dozens of products around designed to deal with cellulite, but to really tackle the problem you should follow a three-pronged approach, combining:

■ Circulation-boosting tactics
■ Diet
■ Exercise

BOOST YOUR CIRCULATION

Here are several ways to boost your circulation and your lymphatic system. Whichever one you choose, aim to follow it for at least five minutes a day.

■ Use a massage glove or rough sisal mitt to stimulate your skin.

Make your own cellulite cream

Some women swear by aromatherapy to treat their cellulite. There are many ready-blended oils on the market, but you can make your own. Just add two drops each of rosemary and fennel essential oils to three teaspoons of carrier oil, such as almond oil. Massage this mixture daily thoroughly into the affected areas.

■ Use a soft body brush on damp or dry skin, brushing in long, sweeping movements over the afflicted area, and working in the direction of the heart.

■ Use a cellulite cream. These usually contain natural ingredients such as horse chestnut and ivy to pep up your circulation. However, you can make them doubly effective by massaging them in with your fingers. Some cellulite creams come with their own plastic or rubber hand-held mitts to help boost the circulation.

■ Some women find that aromatherapy helps to reduce their cellulite. There are many ready-blended oils on the market.

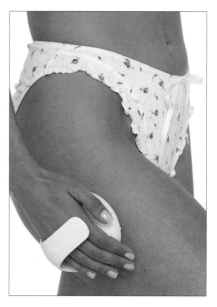

Above: Pep up your circulation and lymphatic system daily to help beat that cellulite.

STEP UP YOUR EXERCISE

Exercise will boost your sluggish circulation and lymphatic system. It will also encourage your body to get rid of the toxins causing your cellulite. Do a regular aerobic workout, exercising for 20-40 minutes, between three and five times a week, and choose from these: brisk walking, jogging, swimming, cycling, tennis, badminton, aerobic classes or running. (It is always wise to consult your doctor before embarking on a new form of exercise.)

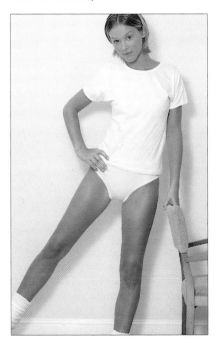

Hip toner

Stand sideways with your hand resting on a chair. Your knees should be slightly bent and your shoulders relaxed. Slowly raise your right leg, keeping your body and raised foot facing forward. Carefully and slowly lower your leg, and then repeat this movement at least 10 times. Then turn round and repeat the exercise with the other leg.

Tone it up!

You can also try these exercises to firm up your legs and give them a better shape. Carried out daily, they will help you win the cellulite battle.

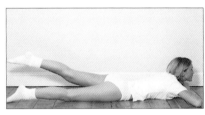

Bottom toner

Lie on your front with your hands on top of one another, resting your chin on them if you wish. Raise one leg about 13 cm (5 in) off the floor, and hold for a count of 10. Bring your leg back to the floor, and repeat 15-20 times with each leg.

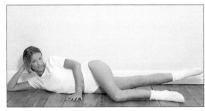

Inner thigh toner

Lie on your side on the floor. With your top leg resting on the floor in front, raise the lower leg off the floor as far as you can without straining, then gently lower it again. Repeat 10 times, then turn over and work the other leg.

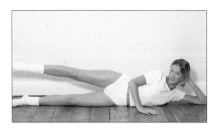

Outer thigh toner

Lie on your side, supporting your head with your hand. Bend your lower leg behind you and tilt your hips slightly forward. Place your other hand on the floor in front of you for balance. Slowly lift your upper leg, then bring it down to touch the lower one, and repeat this action at least six times. Repeat on the other side.

FOLLOW A DETOX DIET

To detoxify your body you need to follow a healthy low-fat, high-fibre diet – one that contains plenty of fresh fruit and vegetables. The great news is, if you have any excess weight to lose it will naturally fall away by following these rules.

■ Eat at least five servings of fresh fruit and vegetables every day.

■ Cut down on the amount of fat you eat. For instance, grill rather than fry foods, and cut off visible fat from meat.

■ Water cleanses your system and flushes toxins from body cells, so drink at least two litres (quarts) of pure water every day.

■ Change from caffeine-laden tea and coffee to herbal teas and decaffeinated coffee. Sip pure fruit juices rather than fizzy drinks.

Brownie Points in the Sun

There's nothing that lifts your spirits like spending time in the sunshine. However, you need to take special care of your skin against the potential dangers of suntanning.

KNOW YOUR SPFs

The initials SPF stand for Sun Protection Factor. The higher the number of the SPF, the more protection the product will give you from the burning ultraviolet B (UVB) rays. To decide which SPF suits you, you need to know how vulnerable your skin is to the sun's UVB rays. Dermatologists divide skins into the following six types.

Skin type 1

Always burns, never tans. Fair-skinned, usually with freckles. Red or blonde hair. Typical Anglo-Saxon or Irish skin type.
UK/North Europe: Total sunblock.
USA/Tropics/Africa: Total sunblock.
Mediterranean: Total sunblock.

Skin type 2

Burns easily and tans with difficulty. Fair hair and pale skin. Typical North European skin type.
UK/North Europe: Start with SPF 20 and use sunblock on delicate areas. Progress gradually to SPF 15.
USA/Tropics/Africa: Start with sunblock and progress gradually to SPF 20.
Mediterranean: Start with SPF 20 and use sunblock on delicate areas. Progress gradually to SPF 15.

Skin type 3

Sometimes burns but tans well. Light brown hair and medium skin-tone. A typical North European skin type.
UK/North Europe: Start with SPF 10 and progress to SPF 8.
USA/Tropics/Africa: Start with SPF 20, moving to SPF 15, then SPF 10.
Mediterranean: Start with SPF 15, moving to SPF 10.

Skin type 4

Occasionally burns but tans easily. Usually with brown hair and eyes, and olive skin. The typical Mediterranean skin type.
UK/North Europe: Start with SPF 8, moving to SPF 6.
USA/Tropics/Africa: Start with SPF 15, moving to SPF 8.
Mediterranean: Start with SPF 10, moving to SPF 6.

Skin type 5

Hardly ever burns and tans easily. Dark eyes, dark hair and olive skin. A typical Middle Eastern or Asian skin type.
UK/North Europe: Use SPF 6.
USA/Tropics/Africa: Start with SPF 8 and move to SPF 6.
Mediterranean: Start SPF 8, and move to SPF 6.

Skin type 6

Almost never burns. Dark hair, eyes, and skin. A typical African or Afro-Caribbean skin type.
UK/North Europe: No sunscreen is needed.
USA/Tropics/Africa: Start with SPF 8 and move to SPF 6.
Mediterranean: Use SPF 6 throughout.

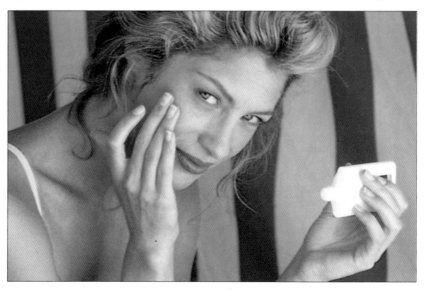

Above: Protect and survive. Guard against ageing and the burning rays of the sun with an effective sun cream.

YOUR SAFE TAN PLAN

■ Apply suntan lotion (block) before you go into the sun and before you dress, to ensure that you don't miss any areas.

■ Gradually build up the time you spend in the sun. Never be tempted to burn – it's a sign of skin damage.

■ Stay out of the sun between 12 noon and 3 o'clock when the sun is at its hottest. Move into the shade or cover up with a T-shirt and broad-brimmed hat.

■ If you're playing a lot of sports or swimming, choose a special sports formula or waterproof formulation.

■ Lips need a good lip screen to protect them from burning and chapping.

■ Like skincare ranges, there are hypoallergenic suncare products around, so ask at your pharmacist.

JOIN THE BROWNIES – WITH A FAKE TAN

The safest tan of all is one that comes out of a bottle. There are three main ways to fake a tan.

Bronzing powders

Use powders on your face in the same way as a blusher. Make sure that the one you use is not too pearlized, or you'll really shimmer in the sunshine.

Wash-off tanners

This is the simplest way to create an instant tan on your face and body. You simply smooth on the cream and then wash it away at the end of the day.

Self tanners

Formulations contain an active ingredient called dihydroxyacetone (DHA), which is absorbed by the surface skin cells and turns brown in the presence of oxygen – which creates the "tan". This process usually takes three to four hours, and the effects last until these skin cells are naturally shed – which can be from a few days up to a week. Self tanners make an acceptable alternative to the real thing.

SELF-TANNING TIPS

■ Use a body scrub first to rub away the dead flaky skin that can soak up colour and create a patchy finish.

■ Massage in plenty of body lotion over the area to be treated. This will combat any remaining dry areas and give a smooth surface on which to apply the tanning lotion.

■ If there's a shade choice, go with the lighter one, because you can always apply a second layer later on.

■ Work the product firmly into the skin until it feels completely dry. Any excess left on the surface is likely to go patchy.

■ If you've applied self tanner to your body, wipe areas that don't normally tan with damp cotton wool pads (cotton balls) – armpits, nipples, soles of feet and fingers. On the face, work the cotton wool around eyebrows, hairline and jawline.

■ While there are self-tanning products that offer some protection from the sun until you wash your skin, it's best to use them in conjunction with the best sunscreen for your skin type.

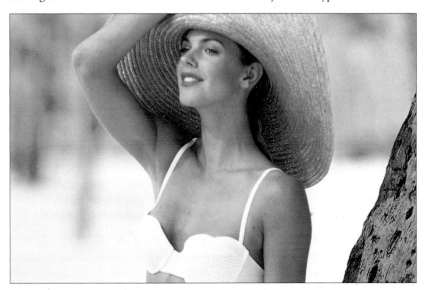

Above: Go for the glow with a light tan.

Your Top Skincare Questions

1 Night watch

Q "My dry skin needs night cream, but I seem to lose most of it onto my pillow. Any solutions?"

A Put a little night cream into the palm of your hand, then gently rub your hands together. The heat created will help liquefy the cream and make it more easily absorbed. Gently massage it into your skin, and you'll find it sinks in better. Another method is to place the cream in a teaspoon, and heat gently over a low gas flame on the cooker until just warm, before applying as usual. It sounds strange, but it really works.

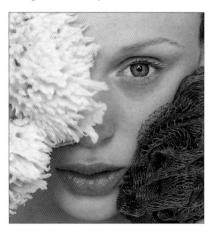

Above: The soft touch of a sponge or facecloth is a cheap – and effective – option to a facial scrub.

2 Polished perfection

Q "I spend a fortune on skincare products, but resent paying for an exfoliator. Are there any alternatives?"

A Yes, here's a good, cheap alternative to facial scrubs. After washing your skin, gently massage with a soft facecloth or natural sponge to ease away the dead surface skin cells that can give your complexion a muddy look. Make sure you avoid ones with scratchy surfaces as they'll be too harsh for your skin. If you have dry skin, massage a little cream cleanser onto damp skin, then rub over the top with your flannel (wash cloth). Rinse afterwards, then apply moisturizer in the normal way. It is essential to wash the facecloth after every couple of uses and to hang it up to dry in between to prevent the build-up of bacteria.

3 Lip tricks

Q "How can I stop my lips from getting so chapped and flaky in winter?"

A This three-step action plan will help.

■ Massage dry lips with a generous dollop of petroleum jelly. Allow it to work for a couple of minutes to soften your skin. Then, gently rub your lips with a warm, damp facecloth. As the petroleum jelly is removed, the flakes of skin will come with it.

■ Smooth your lips morning and night with a lip balm.

■ Switch to a moisturizing lipstick to prevent your lips from drying out during the daytime.

4 Red nose day

Q "It's so embarrassing! My nose looks really red in the winter. What's the best way to cover it?"

A Try smoothing a little green foundation or concealer over the red area before applying your normal foundation and powder. Although it sounds strange, the green works by cancelling out the redness

– leaving your skin looking a normal shade again.

5 Winter sun

Q "Someone told me you should still wear a sunscreen in winter. Is this true?"

A Yes, if you want to guard against the signs of ageing. Exposure to sunlight is thought to be the main cause of wrinkling, and the ultraviolet rays that are responsible for this process are around every single day of the year. You don't, however, need to use a suntan lotion – just choose one of the many moisturizers that contain sunscreens.

6 Lighten up

Q "My skin feels as though it needs a richer cream in the winter months, but I find most of them too heavy. What can you suggest?"

A Choose the level of moisturizer that feels right for you. Just because moisturizer is heavier, it doesn't necessarily mean

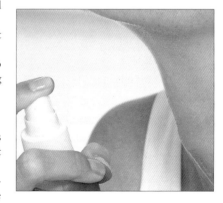

Above: Puttin' on the spritz - boost the moisture in your skin by spraying with water before moisturizing.

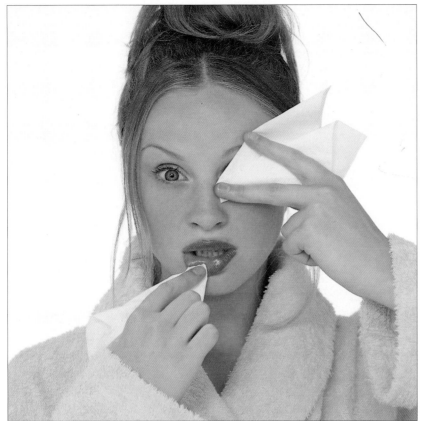

Left: Remove all traces of make-up before going to bed.

8 Sensitive issue

Q "Why does my skin feel more sensitive in winter than summer?"

A Eighty per cent of women claim to have sensitive skin – which tingles, itches and is prone to dryness. It can be aggravated by harsh winter weather, such as the winds and cold, because this breaks down the natural oily layer which protects your skin. Milder summer weather doesn't tend to be so hard on the skin. The best way to cope is to moisturize your skin regularly with a hypoallergenic cream that is specially formulated for sensitive skin.

9 Pregnant pause

Q "I'm pregnant and have developed patches of darker colour on my face, particularly under my eyes and around my mouth. What causes this?"

A This is called chloasma, or "the mask of pregnancy". It's triggered by a change in hormones at this time and is made more obvious by sunbathing. Cover up under the sun and wear a sunblock to prevent the patches from becoming denser. It usually fades within a few months of having your baby. Chloasma can also be triggered by the contraceptive pill, but disappears again once you stop taking them.

10 On the spot

Q "I suffer from oily skin, but find blemish creams too drying. What can you suggest?"

A Many women have skin that has dry patches as well as blemishes. The solution is to choose an antibacterial cream that

it's more effective. You can help seal in extra moisture to your skin by spritzing your complexion with water before applying it. Also, choose a nourishing foundation or tinted moisturizer to ensure that your skin stays smooth and soft all day long. You can help counteract the drying effects of central heating by placing a bowl of water near the radiators to replenish the moisture levels in the air.

7 Water factor

Q "I like the feeling of water on my face, but I find soap too drying. Should I switch to a cream cleanser instead?"

A If you have dry skin, it's generally better to use a creamy cleanser, which you apply with your fingertips and remove with cotton wool pads (cotton balls) or soft tissues. This will prevent too much moisture from being lost from the surface of your skin. However, normal and oily skins can still happily use water – but switch to a facial wash or wash-off cleanser instead. They're specially formulated to be non-drying, while still getting your face clean – and you can splash with water as much as you like!

will kill off the cause of your blemishes, while soothing the skin around them. This means you won't be left with dry patches of skin as well as blemishes.

11 Treatment sprays

Q " I find body lotions too hot and sticky to wear after bathing. Is there anything else I can try?"

A There's a lovely new trend for body treatment sprays, which combine the moisturizing and toning properties of a body care product with the fragrance of a traditional perfume. This means they'll make you smell beautifully fresh as well as lightly moisturize your skin. Many of the large perfume companies now offer a choice of these products.

12 The throat vote

Q "The skin on my neck looks grey and dull. Are there any special treatments I can use?"

A Necks can quickly shown the signs of ageing. This is mainly due to the fact that they have a lack of sebaceous glands. Using a creamy cleanser can help. Massage in, leave to dissolve dirt, and then remove with cotton wool pads (cotton balls). Dull grey skin will benefit from regular exfoliation – scrub briskly with a facecloth or soft shaving brush. Grey lines on the neck and throat can be bleached away by smoothing plain yogurt over clean skin. Leave on for about half an hour, then rinse away thoroughly with warm water. Boost softness by smoothing on moisturizer. Your ordinary cream moisturizer will do the job.

13 Beautiful back

Q "How can I get rid of the pimples on my back and bottom?"

A Because backs are covered up and hard to reach, they're prone to breakouts. Keep yours blemish free by exfoliating daily with a loofah or body brush to remove dry, flaking skin and superficial blemishes. For more stubborn pimples, try a clay mask to draw out deep-seated impurities. Smooth onto broken-out areas, leave until dry, then rinse away with lots of warm water.

14 Mole watch

Q "I understand you need to keep an eye on moles on your skin to guard against the risk of skin cancer. But what exactly should I be looking for?"

A Moles are clumps of clustered pigment cells that are nearly always darker than freckles. All changes in existing moles

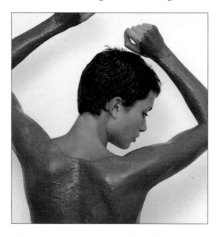

Above: Back to basics with a clay mask for the body.

should be checked by your doctor. Any that cause concern will be removed and sent off for analysis. You should also check moles yourself once a month. Try the following ABCD Code: check for A

(asymmetry); B (border irregularity); C (colour change); D (change in diameter).

15 Shadow sense

Q "I've got dark shadows under my eyes. What's the best way to deal with them?"

A Dark shadows can be the result of a variety of causes, including fatigue, anaemia, poor digestion and lack of fresh air. They can also be hereditary. If in doubt, consult your doctor for advice. Take steps to ensure that you're cutting out the causes – for instance, getting a good night's sleep and keeping to a low-fat, high-fibre diet.

For special occasions, you can bathe the area with pads soaked in ice-cold water for 15 minutes. This will help lessen the shadow effect temporarily. Or cover shadows by dotting on some concealer over the affected area.

16 Brown baby

Q "Is there anything I can do to hang on to my tan for longer?"

A Just when you want to show off a golden tan, it begins to peel away. This is because your skin is especially dry after sunbathing, so it sheds its old cells more quickly. You can prolong the colour for a little while longer by applying lots of body lotion in the morning and evening. Apply it while your skin is still damp to make it extra effective. Apply a little fake tan every few days to keep your colour topped up. Or better still - protect your skin by not tanning at all.

17 Sticky situation

Q "I exercise a lot and find body odour a problem. How can I prevent it?"

A Sweating is your body's natural cooling device. Sweat itself has no odour, but it begins to smell when it comes into contact with bacteria on the skin's surface. Keeping underarms hair-free can help prevent sweat from being trapped.

Opt for an antiperspirant deodorant rather than just an ordinary deodorant alone. The antiperspirants help prevent sweating, while the deodorant helps prevent odour. As a result, a product with the combination of the two is highly effective. Also, try to wear natural fibres next to your skin because they help you to stay fresh for longer.

18 Massage magic

Q "I had a facial massage in a beauty salon. Is there a way I can give myself one at home?"

A Yes, just like every other part of your body, your face will look better after a bit of exercise, and a massage is the ideal way to give your complexion a workout. Pour a few drops of vegetable oil into the palms of your hands and smooth it onto your face and neck. Make sure your skin is damp, as this makes the oil go on more easily. Then follow these steps:

■ Use your fingers to stroke upwards from the base of your neck to your chin.

■ Continue with long strokes up one side of your face, then the other.

■ Now go around your nose and up towards your forehead.

■ When you get to your forehead, stroke it across from left to right using one hand. Finish off by gently drawing a circle around each eye using one finger.

19 Stretch marks

Q "Is there anything I can do to get rid of the stretch marks that have appeared on my tummy, breasts and thighs?"

A There's little you can do once you've got them, except wait until they start to fade. However, keeping your skin well moisturized can help guard against getting them in the first place. An application of fake tan can be a good disguise for stretch marks that might be on view.

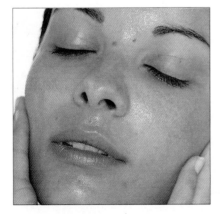

Above: Stroke away the strains and stresses of the day.

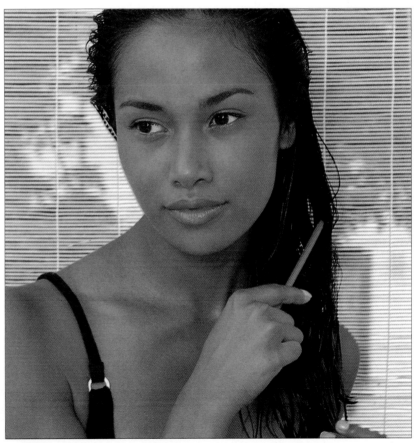

Above: Take time in the bathroom to pamper yourself from head to toe.

Beauty Buzzwords

If you're confused about the various claims and ingredients in your skincare products, check out what they mean here in your guide to the most commonly found skincare jargon.

Allergy-screened

Means that the individual ingredients in the product have gone through exacting tests to ensure that they're safe to use and that there's just the minimum risk of causing allergy.

Aloe vera

The juice from the leaves of this cactus-type plant is often used in skincare ingredients because of its soothing, protecting and moisturizing qualities.

Antioxidants

Work by mopping up and absorbing "free radicals" (highly reactive molecules that can damage your skin and cause premature ageing) from your skin. Good antioxidants are the ACE vitamins, i.e. vitamins A, C and E.

Benzoyl peroxide

An ingredient commonly used in over-the-counter spot and acne treatments. It gently peels surface skin and unclogs blocked follicles which can cause spots.

Cocoa butter

Comes from the seeds of the cacao tree in tropical climates. Cocoa butter is an excellent moisturizer, especially for dry skin on the body.

Right: A pH balanced facial wash will help prevent your skin feeling tight.

Collagen

An elastic type of substance in the underlying tissues of your skin that provide support and springiness. Collagen is a popular ingredient in skincare treatments, although it's doubtful if a molecule this size can actually penetrate the skin.

Dermatologically tested

Means the product has been patch tested on a panel of human volunteers to monitor it for any tendency to cause irritation. This means it's usually suitable for sensitive skins.

Elastin

Fibres in the underlying layer of your skin, rather like collagen, which help give it strength and elasticity.

Exfoliation

The whisking away of the top layers of dead surface cells from your skin, making it look brighter and feel smoother.

Fruit acids

These are also known as AHAs or alpha-hydroxy acids. They're commonly found in natural products, such as fruit, sour milk and wine. AHAs are included in many face creams because they work by breaking down the protein bonds that hold together the dead cells on the skin's surface, to reveal newer, fresher skin underneath.

Humectants

Are ingredients often found in moisturizers, as they work by attracting moisture to themselves, and so keep the surface layers of your skin well hydrated.

Hypoallergenic

These products are usually fragrance-free, contain the minimum of colouring agents and no known irritants or sensitizers. This is not a total guarantee that no one will have an allergic reaction to them. Some people are allergic to water.

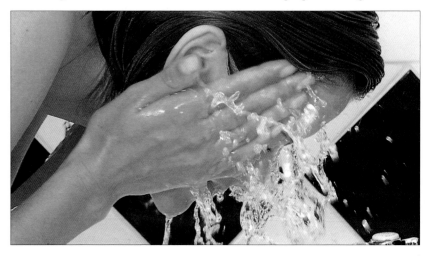

Jojoba oil

A gentle, non-irritant oil which makes an excellent moisturizer as it is easily absorbed into the skin and helps improve the condition of the hair and scalp.

Lanolin free

Means a product doesn't contain anolin. At one time it was thought that lanolin was a skin allergen, although evidence now seems to show that lanolin is even suitable for sensitive skins.

Liposomes

Tiny fluid-filled spheres of the same material that forms cell membranes. Their very small size is said to let them penetrate into the skin's living cells, where they act as delivery parcels that release their active ingredients.

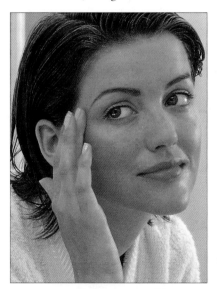

Above: Ensure your moisturizer has an effective sunscreen – check the SPF rating to be sure.

Milia

Another word for whiteheads – small pimples on the skin. Oil produced from the sebaceous glands gathers to form a white plug that is trapped under the skin. You can try to remove these by gently squeezing with tissue-covered fingers or treat them with an antibacterial cream.

Non-comedogenic

Means the product has been screened to eliminate ingredients which can clog the follicles and encourage blackheads and spots (a comedo is a blackhead). It's particularly useful for oily skins.

Oil of Evening Primrose

It is very useful for helping your skin retain its moisture. It's a wonderful moisturizer, particularly for dry or very dry skins, as it hydrates, protects and soothes. Many sufferers of eczema find it useful.

pH balanced

Refers to the pH scale, which measures the acidity or alkalinity of a solution. Seven means that it is neutral. Any number below that is acidic, and numbers above are alkaline. Healthy skin has a slightly acidic reading, so pH balanced skincare products are slightly acidic to maintain this natural optimum level.

SPF

Stands for Sun Protection Factor. It tells you how long the sun cream or moisturizer will protect you from the sun's ultraviolet B (UVB) rays. The higher the number, the more protection it gives you.

T-zone

The T-zone is the area across the forehead and down the centre of the face where the oil glands and sweat glands of the face are most concentrated.

Ultraviolet (UV) rays

UVB rays will burn and damage your skin if you sunbathe too long. UVA rays are strong all year round and cause ageing and wrinkling of the skin. Guard against this with a broad-spectrum sun cream, which contains both UVA and UVB filters to protect you year round.

Vitamin E

Often used in moisturizers because it can help combat dryness and the signs of ageing. It's also useful for helping to heal scars and burns.

Water soluble

Cleansers are described as water soluble when they contain oils to dissolve grime and make-up from the skin. They have the added bonus that they can be easily rinsed away from the skin with plenty of fresh, clean water.

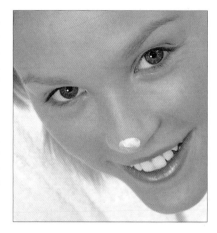

Above: Try the healing benefits of vitamin E on your skin.

Healthy Hair

Beautiful, shining hair is a valuable asset.
It can also be a versatile fashion accessory,
to be coloured, curled, dressed up or smoothed
down – all in a matter of minutes. However, too
much attention combined with the effects of a poor
diet, pollution, air-conditioning and central heating
can mean that your hair becomes the bane of your
life rather than your crowning glory. A daily haircare
routine and prompt treatment when problems do
arise are of vital importance in maintaining
the natural beauty of healthy hair.

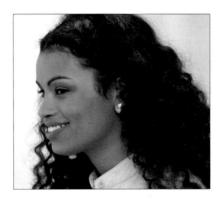

Above: Individual hair types need
individual treatments: adopt a personal
routine to keep your hair at its best.

Right: Healthy hair reflects well-being
and has a natural beauty of its own.

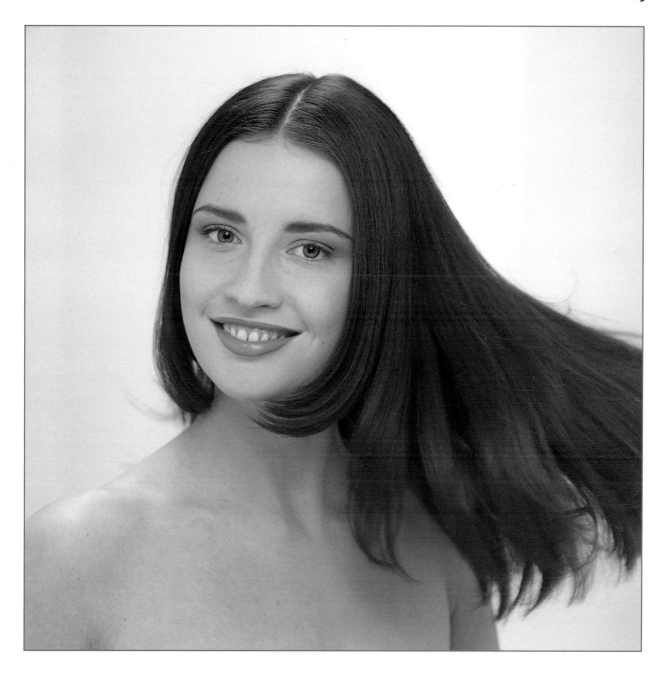

What is Hair?

Human hair is made up of a protein called keratin, as well as some moisture and the trace metals and minerals found in the rest of the body. The visible part of the hair is called the shaft and is in fact dead tissue: the only living part of the hair is its root, the dermal papilla, which lies below the surface of the scalp in a depression known as the follicle. The dermal papilla is made up of cells that are fed by the bloodstream.

Each hair consists of three layers. The outer layer, or cuticle, is the hair's protective shield and has tiny overlapping scales. When the cuticle scales lie flat, the hair feels soft and looks glossy. If the cuticle scales have been damaged, the hair will be dull and brittle and will tangle easily.

Beneath the cuticle lies the cortex, which give hair strength and elasticity. The cortex also contains the pigment melanin, which gives hair its natural colour. At the centre of each hair is the

Below: Spring forward for great hair!

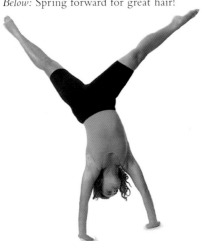

medulla, which is believed to supply the cortex and cuticle with nutrients.

Hair's natural shine is supplied by sebum, a conditioning oil composed of waxes and fats, which also contains a natural antiseptic to help fight infection. Sebum is produced by the sebaceous glands present in the dermis. The glands release sebum into the hair follicles. Sebum gives a protective coating to the hair shaft, smoothing the cuticle scales and helping hair retain moisture and elasticity. When the sebaceous glands produce too much sebum the result is greasy hair. Conversely, if too little sebum is produced the hair will be dry.

THE GROWTH CYCLE

The only living part of hair is underneath the scalp – when the hair has grown through the scalp it is dead tissue. There are three stages of hair growth: the anagen phase with active growth; the catagen, or transitional, phase when growth stops but cell activity continues; and the telogen phase, when all activity stops. When there is no further growth, the old hair is pushed out by the new growth and the cycle begins again.

Below: A sensible fitness plan means a boost to your health – and your hair.

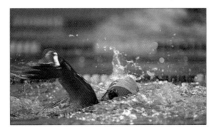

THE IMPORTANCE OF DIET

Like the rest of the body, healthy hair depends on a good diet to ensure it is supplied with all the nutrients it needs. However, if you eat a balanced diet with plenty of fresh ingredients you shouldn't need to take any supplementary vitamins to promote healthy hair growth.

An adequate supply of protein in the diet is essential to healthy hair. Good sources of protein include lean meat, poultry, fish, cheese and eggs as well as nuts, seeds and pulses. Fish, seaweed, nuts, yogurt and cottage cheese will all give hair strength and a natural shine. Wholegrain foods help in the formation of keratin, the major component of hair. Try to eat at least three pieces of fruit a day – it is packed with fibre, vitamins and minerals. Avoid saturated fat, which is found in red meat, fried foods and dairy products. Choose skimmed or semi-skimmed milk and low-fat cheese and yogurt, and substitute vegetable oils such as olive oil for animal fats.

Below: Silky hair is a real beauty asset!

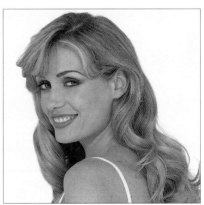

PROMOTING HEALTHY HAIR

■ Cut down on tea and coffee – they are powerful stimulants, increasing the excretion of water and nutrients and hampering the absorption of minerals. Drink between six and eight glasses of mineral water a day, along with herbal teas and unsweetened fruit juices.

■ Alcohol dilates blood vessels and increases blood flow to the tissues but is antagonistic to the nutrients vital for healthy hair, so limit yourself to an occasional drink.

■ Regular exercise stimulates the blood circulation, encouraging a supply of nutrients to the hair root.

Fact File

■ Hair grows about 1 cm/1/2 in per month.
■ A single strand of hair "lives" for up to seven years.
■ If a person never had their hair cut it would grow to a length of approximately 107 cm/42 in before falling out.
■ Women have more hair than men.
■ Hair grows faster in the summer months and during sleep.
■ Hair grows fastest between the ages of 16 and 24.

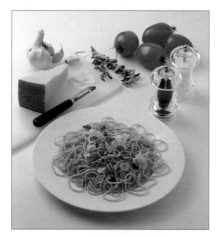

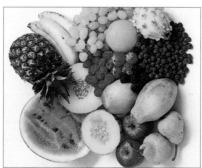

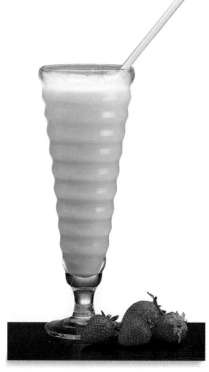

COLOUR

Hair colour is closely related to skin colour and is governed by the same pigment, melanin. The number of melanin granules in the cortex of the hair and the shape of the granules will determine a person's natural hair colour.

For most people the melanin granules are elongated in shape. People who have a large number of elongated melanin granules in the cortex have black hair, those with slightly fewer elongated granules have brown hair, and people with even less will be blonde. When the melanin granules are spherical or oval in shape the hair will appear red.

If spherical or oval granules appear in combination with a small number of elongated ones, then the hair will have rich, reddish-brown tinges. If spherical granules combine with a large number of elongated granules then the blackness of the hair will mask the redness, giving just a subtle tinge to the hair.

Hair colour darkens with age, but at some stage during middle-age the pigment formation slows down and silvery-grey hairs begin to appear. Gradually, the production of melanin ceases, and all the hair becomes colourless – or what is generally termed grey. When melanin granules are completely lacking from birth, as in albinos, the hair appears pure white.

Far left: Swap tea and coffee for healthy unsweetened fruit juices.

Above left: A balanced diet will supply all the nutrients you need for healthy hair.

Left: Eat lots of fresh fruit to help keep your hair shiny and soft.

Texture and Type

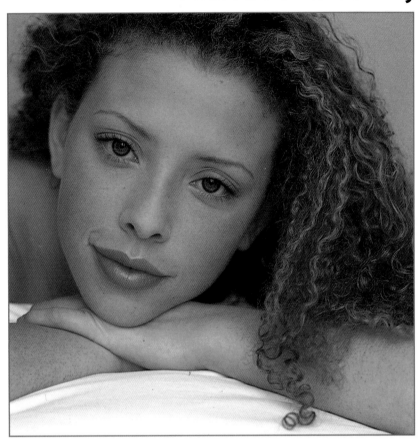

Left: Knowing your hair type is an important part of caring for your hair.

The texture of your hair is determined by the size and shape of the hair follicles, which is a genetic trait controlled by hormones and related to age and racial characteristics.

Whether hair is curly, wavy, or straight depends on two things: its shape as it grows out of the follicle and the distribution of keratin-producing cells at the roots. If viewed in cross-section, straight hair tends to be round, wavy hair tends to be oval, and curly hair kidney-shaped.

Straight hair is formed by roots that produce the same number of keratin cells around the follicle. In curly hair the production of keratin cells is uneven, so that there are more cells on one side of the oval-shaped follicle than on the other. Furthermore, the production of excess cells alternates between the sides, causing the developing hair to grow first in one direction and then in the other. The result of an imbalance in cell production will be curly hair.

The natural colour of the hair also affects the texture. Natural blondes have finer hair than brunettes while redheads have the thickest hair.

Hair can be divided into three categories: fine, medium, and coarse and thick. Fine hair can be strong or weak but, because of its texture, all fine hair lacks volume. Medium hair is neither thick nor thin and is strong and elastic. Thick and coarse hair is abundant and heavy, with a tendency to grow outwards from the scalp as well as downwards.

A single head of hair may consist of several different textures. Fine hair is found on the temples, hairline and at the nape of the head, while the texture over the rest of the head may be medium or even coarse.

DRY, NORMAL OR GREASY?

Hair type is determined by the amount of sebum the body produces. Treatment programmes such as perming, colouring, and heat styling will also have an effect on hair type, and sometimes the effects of these will be permanent. The different hair types are described below, together with advice on haircare.

Dry hair

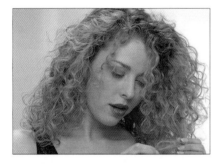

Hair that is too dry looks dull, feels dry, tangles easily and is difficult to comb or brush. It is often thick at the roots but thinner, and sometimes split, at the ends. **Causes** Excessive shampooing, overuse of heat-styling equipment, misuse of colour or perms, damage from the sun or harsh weather conditions. These factors deplete the moisture content of hair so that it loses its elasticity, bounce and suppleness. Dryness can also be the result of a sebum deficiency on the hair's surface, caused by a lack of or decrease in sebaceous gland secretions. **Solutions** Use a nourishing shampoo and an intensive conditioner specifically for dry hair. Treat the hair as gently as you can: allow hair to dry naturally whenever possible. Consider having a trim if you have split ends.

Normal hair

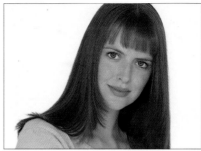

Normal hair is neither greasy nor dry, has not been permed or coloured, holds its style and looks good most of the time.

Greasy hair

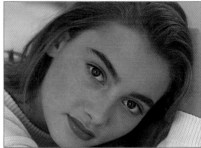

This looks lank and oily and is often unmanageable. It needs frequent washing. **Causes** Overproduction of sebum as a result of hormone disturbances, stress, excessive brushing, perspiration or a diet rich in saturated fat. **Solutions** Use a gentle shampoo that also gives the hair volume. A light perm will lift the hair at the roots and limit the dispersal of sebum. Rethink your diet: reduce dairy fats and greasy foods. Eat plenty of fresh foods, and drink six to eight glasses of water every day.

Combination hair

Combination hair is greasy at the roots but dry and sometimes split at the ends. **Causes** Chemical treatments, overuse of detergent-based shampoos, overexposure to sunlight and overuse of heat styling equipment. Repeated abuse provokes a reaction in sebum secretion at the roots and an alteration in the scales, which can no longer fulfil their protective role. As a result, the hair ends become dry. **Solutions** Use only gentle products on the hair. Formulations for oily hair and for dry hair may contribute to the problem, so use a product designed for combination hair. If this is not possible try using a shampoo for oily hair and finish by applying a conditioner only from the middle lengths to the ends of the hair.

Coloured or permed hair

Hair that has been coloured or permed is often more porous than untreated hair and needs careful handling, using gentle cleansers and quality conditioners. Colour-care products help to prevent fading by protecting the hair from sunlight. Specialist products for permed hair help maintain elasticity.

Below: Clever haircare means great hair.

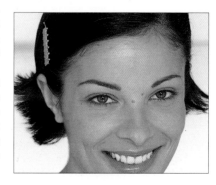

The Cut

Hair growth varies over different parts of the head. This is why your cut can appear to be out of shape very quickly.

As a general rule, a short precision cut needs trimming every four weeks, a longer style every six to eight weeks.

Even if you want to grow your hair you should have it trimmed at least every three months to prevent splitting.

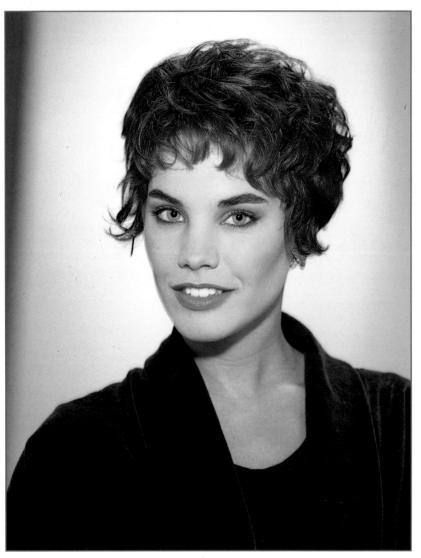

Hairdressers use a variety of techniques and tools to make hair appear thicker, fuller, straighter or curlier, according to the desired effect. The techniques and tools they use are explained below.

Blunt cutting

This is when the ends are cut straight across; it is often used for hair of one length and for fine hair. The weight and fullness of the hair is distributed around the perimeter of the shape.

Clippers

Clippers are used for close-cut styles and sometimes to finish off a cut. Shaved clipper cuts need to be trimmed very regularly to keep the style.

Graduated hair

Graduated hair is cut at an angle to give lots of fullness on top and to gradually blend the top hair into shorter lengths at the nape.

Layering

Layering the hair evenly distributes the weight and fullness, giving a soft and round appearance to the style.

Left: This permed style was cut into a short crop with heavy layers. The hair was diffuser-dried to give extra movement, then sculpting gel was used to emphasize the side kicks and styling lotion was added for a textured look.

Slide cutting

This technique (also called slithering or feathering) thins the hair. Scissors are used in a sliding action, backwards and forwards along the hair length, often when the hair is dry.

Razor cutting

Razor cutting creates softness, tapering and internal movement so that the hair moves more freely. It can also be used to shorten hair. Thinning hair, either with thinning scissors or a razor, removes bulk and weight without affecting the overall length of the hair.

CLEVER CUTS

■ Fine, thin, flyaway hair can be given extra volume and movement by blunt cutting. Mid-length hair can be given volume, while short, thin hair can have the edges graduated to give movement.

■ Fine hair can also be razor cut for a thicker and more voluminous effect. Do not let fine hair grow long. As soon as it reaches the shoulders it can look wispy.

■ Thick hair can be controlled by reducing the weight to give more style and direction. Avoid very short styles because the hair will tend to stick out. Try a layered cut with added movement.

■ Layering the hair also helps achieve height and eliminate weight. On shorter styles the weight can be reduced with thinning scissors used on the ends only.

■ Hair can grow in different directions, causing styling problems. For example, a cowlick is normally found on the front hairline and occurs when the hair grows

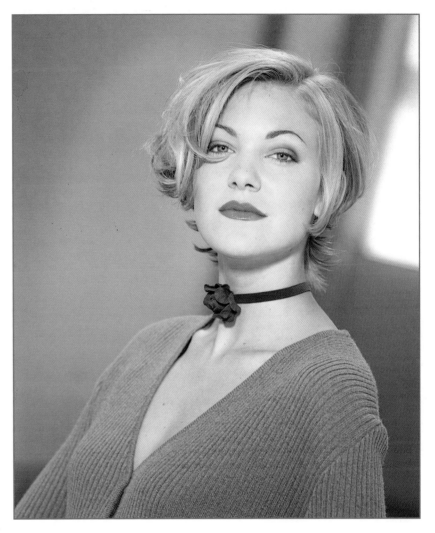

in a swirl, backwards and then forwards. Clever cutting can redistribute the weight and go some way towards solving the problem. For a double crown – when there are two pivots of hair, rather than the usual one – choose a style which gives height at the crown.

Above: For this sleek seventies look, extra body was given to fine hair with a razor cut to create movement. The hair was blow-dried using a large round brush to pull the hair straight. Finally, sculpting wax was used to give maximum smoothness and shine.

Shampoo Success

Shampoos are designed to cleanse the hair and scalp, removing dirt and grime without stripping away too much of the natural sebum. They contain cleansing agents, perfume, preservatives and conditioning agents that can coat the hair shaft to make the hair appear thicker. The conditioning agents smooth the cuticle scales so the hair doesn't tangle and help to eliminate static electricity from the hair when it dries.

THE pH FACTOR

The letters pH refer to the acid/alkaline level of a substance. It is calculated on a scale of 1 to 14. Numbers below 7 denote acidity, those over 7 alkalinity. Most shampoos range between a pH factor of 5 and 7; medicated varieties have a pH of about 7.3, which is near neutral. Sebum has a pH factor of between 4.5 and 5.5, which is mildly acidic. Bacteria cannot survive in this pH, and maintaining this protective layer keeps the scalp and hair at their best.

Below: Choose your shampoo carefully.

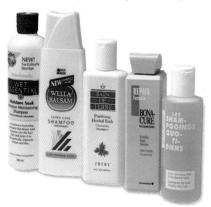

SHAMPOO TIPS

■ Always use the correct shampoo for your hair type.

■ Don't wash your hair in washing-up liquid or soap; they are highly alkaline and will upset your hair's natural pH balance by stripping out the natural oils.

■ Always read the instructions first: some shampoos need to be left on the scalp for a few minutes before rinsing.

■ Buy small sachets of shampoo to test which brand is most suitable for you.

■ Don't wash your hair in the bath; dirty bath water is not conducive to clean hair, and it is difficult to rinse properly without a shower attachment or separate jug.

■ Always wash your brush and comb when you shampoo your hair.

■ Change your shampoo approximately every two weeks; hair develops a resistance to certain ingredients after time.

■ Don't throw away a shampoo that doesn't lather. The amount of suds are determined by the active level of detergent, as well as by the hardness of the water in your area.

■ Many shampoos are labelled "pH balanced", and this means they have the same acidity level as hair. Use a shampoo of this type if you have permed or coloured hair. These shampoos are not necessary for normal hair, as long as you condition your hair after shampooing.

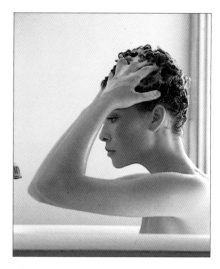

Above: If you wash your hair regularly use a mild shampoo.

Below: Rinse your hair with warm water after shampooing. Continue to rinse until the water runs clear and clean.

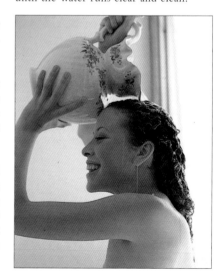

GETTING IT RIGHT

■ Always use a product formulated for your particular hair type, and before shampooing brush your hair to free any tangles and loosen dirt and dead skin cells.

■ Use lukewarm water, as hot water can be uncomfortable on the scalp. Wet the hair, then apply a small amount of shampoo and massage into the roots, using the pads of your fingertips; never use your nails. Pay attention to the hairline area, where make-up and dirt become trapped. Don't rub vigorously or you will stretch the hair.

■ After shampooing, rinse thoroughly until the water runs clean and clear. Repeat only if you think your hair needs it. Blot the hair with a clean towel to remove excess water.

MASSAGING THE SCALP

Massage helps maintain a healthy scalp by improving the circulation and delivering nutrients and oxygen to the hair follicle. It also helps loosen dead skin cells and can redress the overproduction of sebum, which makes hair greasy.

You can give yourself a scalp massage at home. Use warm olive oil if the scalp is dry or tight. Try equal parts of witch hazel and mineral water if you have an oily scalp. For a normal scalp, use equal parts rose and mineral waters.

■ Begin the massage by gently rotating your scalp using the tips of your fingers, taking care not to use your nails. Start the massage at the forehead, move across to the sides and then work over the crown to the nape of the neck. Try to keep the movement continuous.

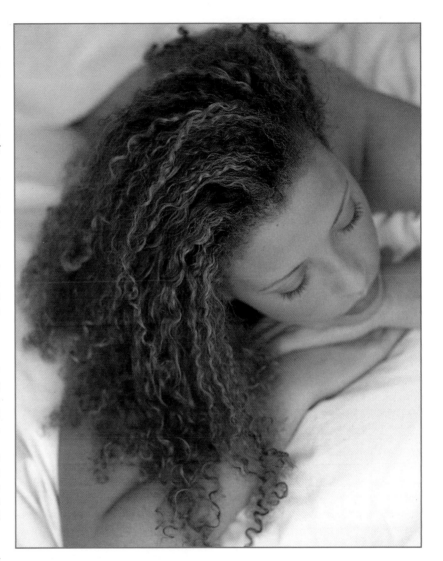

■ Next, place your fingertips firmly on your scalp without exerting too much pressure. Push your fingers together, then pull them apart through the hair in a gentle kneading motion, without lifting or moving them.

■ Massage for a minute, then move to the next section. Treat your entire scalp and upper neck in this way.

Above: Healthy, shiny hair looks great and reflects good physical well-being.

Getting into Condition

Few people are able to wash their hair and let the matter rest at that; most need help just to overcome the effects of modern living, not to mention the occasional problem that needs treatment. Here is a guide to the range of products available to get hair back into condition.

THE CONDITIONERS

Glossy hair has cuticle scales that lie flat and neatly overlap, reflecting the light. Perming and colouring, rough handling and heat styling all conspire to lift the cuticles, allowing moisture to be lost from the cortex and making hair dry, lacklustre, and prone to tangles. Severely damaged cuticles break off completely, which means that the hair gets thinner and eventually breaks.

To put the shine back into hair it may be necessary to use a specific conditioner that meets the hair's requirements. Conditioners, with the exception of hot oils, should be applied to freshly shampooed hair that has first been blotted dry with a clean towel to remove the excess moisture.

Basic conditioners

These coat the hair with a fine film, temporarily smoothing down the cuticle and making the hair glossier and easier to manage. Leave for a few minutes before rinsing thoroughly.

Conditioning sprays

These are used prior to styling and form a protective barrier against the harmful effects of heat. They are also good for reducing static electricity on flyaway hair.

Hot oils

These give an intensive, deep nourishing treatment. To use, place the unopened tube in a cup of hot water and leave for one minute. Wet the hair and towel it dry. Massage the hot oil evenly into the scalp and hair. For a more intensive treatment, cover the head with a shower cap. To finish, rinse the hair and shampoo.

Intensive conditioners

These help hair to replenish its natural moisture balance. Use this type if the hair is split, dry, frizzy or difficult to manage. Distribute the conditioner through the hair and allow it to penetrate for two to five minutes. Rinse well with fresh water, lifting your hair from the scalp to wash away any residue.

Below: Condition when and where your hair needs it, not just for the sake of it.

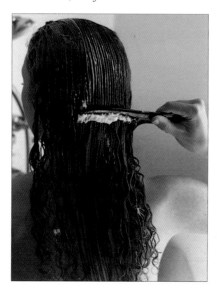

Leave-in conditioners

These are designed to help retain moisture, reduce static and add shine. They are especially good for fine hair as they avoid conditioner overload, which can cause lankness. Convenient and easy-to-use, they also provide a protective barrier against the effects of heat styling. Apply after shampooing but don't rinse off. These products are ideal for daily use.

Restructurants

Restructurants penetrate the cortex, helping to repair and strengthen the inner part of damaged hair. They are helpful if the hair is lank and limp and has lost its natural elasticity as a result of chemical treatments or physical damage.

Split end treatments/serums

Split end treatments and serums condition damaged hair. The best course of action for split ends is to have the ends trimmed, but this does not always solve the whole problem because the hair tends to break off and split at different levels. As an intermediate solution, split ends can be temporarily sealed using specialist conditioners. They are worked into the ends of newly washed hair so that they surround the hair with a microscopic film that leaves the hair shaft smoother.

Colour/perm conditioners

Conditioners for coloured or permed hair are specially designed for chemically treated hair. After-colour products add a protective film around porous areas of the hair, preventing colour loss. After-perm products help stabilize the hair and help to keep the bounce in the curl.

PROBLEMS AND SOLUTIONS

The following hair problems are easily overcome with an appropriate treatment.

Dandruff

Dandruff consists of scaly particles with an oily sheen that lie close to the root.
Causes Poor diet, sluggish metabolism, stress, hormonal imbalance or infection can all increase cell renewal on the scalp, meaning an increase in sebum. The scales will absorb some of the excess oil, but the problem will worsen unless treated.
Solutions Brush the hair before shampooing, using a mild anti-dandruff shampoo to loosen the scales. Follow with a treatment lotion. Avoid excessive use of heat stylers. If the problem persists, consult your family doctor.

Flaky/itchy scalp

This produces tiny pieces of dead skin that flake off the scalp. The scalp can be red or itchy, and the hair looks dull.

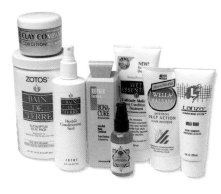

Above: The range of conditioning products now available means that hair problems can be a thing of the past.

Causes Hereditary traits, stress, shampoo residues caused by insufficient rinsing, lack of sebum, harsh shampoos, air conditioning, pollution and central heating.
Solutions Choose a moisturizing shampoo and use a conditioner with herbal extracts to help soothe the scalp.

Fine hair

Fine hair tends to be limp, looks flat and does not hold a style.
Causes The texture is hereditary, but the problem is often made worse by using too heavy a conditioner, which weighs the hair down. Excessive use of styling products can have the same effect.
Solutions Wash the hair with a mild shampoo and use a light conditioner. Volumizing shampoos can help give body, and soft perms will make the hair appear thicker and the style fuller.

Frizzy hair

Frizzy hair results from air moisture being absorbed into the hair. The hair looks dry and lacklustre, and is difficult to control.
Causes Can be inherited or caused by rough treatment, such as too much harsh brushing or pulling the hair into bands.
Solutions When washing the hair, massage the shampoo into the roots and allow the lather to work to the ends. Apply a conditioner from the mid-length of the hair to the ends, or use a leave-in conditioner. The hair is best styled with gel, applied when the hair is wet. The hair can also be dried naturally.

Split ends

Split ends occur when the cuticle is damaged and the fibres of the cortex unravel. The hair is dry, brittle and prone to tangling and can be split at the end.

Causes Over-perming or colouring, insufficient conditioning or too much brushing or backcombing. Careless use of rollers and hairpins, excessive heat styling and not having a regular trim.
Solutions Split ends can't be mended; the only long-term cure is to have them snipped off. What is lost in the length will be gained in quality. Shampoo less often and never use a dryer too near the hair or set it on too high a temperature. Try conditioners and serums that are designed to temporarily seal split ends and give resistance to further splitting.

Product build-up

This is the residue of styling products left on the hair shaft.
Causes Residues combine with mineral deposits in the water and a build-up occurs. The hair is difficult to perm or colour because of a barrier preventing the chemicals from penetrating the hair.
Solutions Use a stripping or clarifying shampoo specially designed to remove product build-up. This is particularly important prior to perming or colouring.

Below: Your hair needs careful handling if it is to look its best!

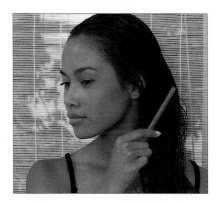

Colouring and Bleaching

Hair colourants have never been better than those available today; nowadays it is a simple matter to add a temporary tone and gloss to the hair or even to make a more permanent change. And there is a wide choice of home colouring products if you like the idea of experimenting yourself.

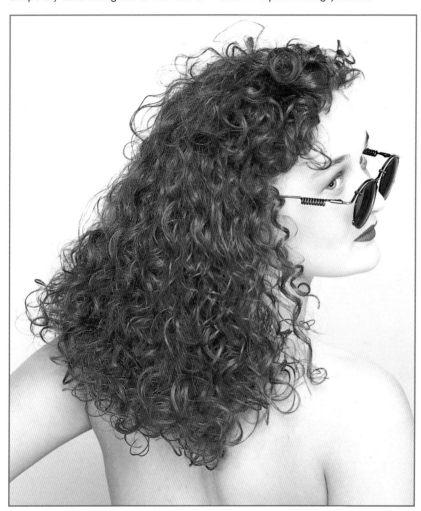

Above: Adding colour to your hair swells the hair and makes it look thicker, and this in turn adds texture and gives the appearance of a healthy head of hair.

Fact File

■ Colouring swells the hair shaft, making fine hair appear thicker.
■ Because colour changes the porosity of the hair it can help combat greasiness.
■ Rich tones reflect more light and give hair a thicker appearance.
■ Highlights give fine hair extra texture and break up the heaviness of very thick hair.
■ Too light a hair colour can make the hair appear thinner.

THE CHOICE

There is a wide range of colouring products available and it helps to know what is on offer before you decide.

Temporary colours

These are usually water-based and are applied to pre-shampooed, wet hair. They work by coating the outside, or cuticle layer, of the hair. The colour washes away in the next shampoo.

Colour setting

Colour setting lotions combine a colour that washes out with a strong setting lotion. They are similar to temporary colours and are perfect for adding tone to grey, white or bleached hair.

Semi-permanent colours

These give a more noticeable effect that lasts for six to eight shampoos. They can only add, enrich, or darken hair colour, they cannot make it any lighter. These colours penetrate the cuticle and coat the outer edge of the cortex. The colour fades gradually and is ideal for those who just want to experiment. Longer lasting semi-permanent colours remain in the hair for 12–20 shampoos. The colour penetrates deeper into the cortex than in semi-permanent colour. This type is perfect for a more lasting change.

Permanent colours

These can be used to lighten or darken hair permanently. The colour is absorbed by the cortex in around 30 minutes, and after this time oxygen in the developer swells the pigments in the colourant and holds them in. The roots may need retouching every six weeks. When retouching it is important to colour only the new hair growth. If the new colour overlaps previously treated hair there will be a build-up of colour from the mid-lengths to the ends, which will make the hair more porous.

NATURAL COLOURING

Vegetable colourants such as henna and chamomile have been used since ancient times to colour hair. Henna is the most widely used natural dye, but colourants can be extracted from a wide variety of plants, including marigold petals, cloves, rhubarb stalks and even tea leaves.

Natural dyes work in the same way as semi-permanent colourants by staining the outside of the hair. However, results are variable and a residue is often left behind, making further colouring with permanent tints or bleaches inadvisable.

Right: Gentle natural colourants, containing herbs and minerals, are available for adding tone and shine.

Henna

Henna enhances natural highlights and makes colour appear richer. The colour fades gradually but frequent applications will give a stronger, longer-lasting effect.

The result that is achieved when using henna depends on the natural colour of the hair. On brunette or black hair it produces a lovely reddish glow, while lighter hair becomes a beautiful titian. Henna is not suitable for use on blonde hair, and on hair that is more than 20 per cent tinted, bleached or highlighted, the resultant colour will be orange.

Always test the henna you intend to use on a few loose hairs (the ones in your hairbrush will do), making a note of the length of time it takes to produce the result you want.

Use neutral henna to add gloss without adding colour. Mix henna and water to a stiff paste. Stir in an egg yolk and a little milk, and mix. Apply to the hair and leave for an hour before rinsing. Repeat every two months.

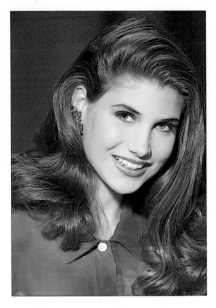

Above: Colour-treated hair needs extra care if it is to really shine! Pay close attention to the look and feel of your hair so that you can be ready to respond straight away if problems occur.

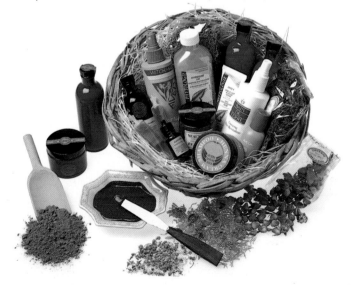

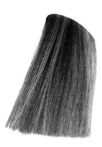

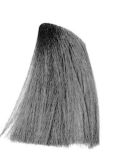

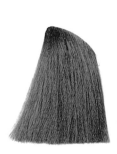

Do's and Don'ts

■ Do rinse henna paste thoroughly or the hair and scalp will feel gritty.

■ Don't expose hennaed hair to strong sunlight, and rinse salt and chlorine from the hair immediately after swimming.

■ Do use a henna shampoo between colour applications to enhance the tone.

■ Don't use shampoos and conditioners containing henna on blonde, grey or chemically treated hair.

■ Do use the same henna product each time you apply henna.

■ Don't use compound henna (with added metallic salts); it can cause long-term hair colouring problems.

Chamomile

Chamomile has a gentle lightening effect on hair and is good for sun-streaking blonde and light brown hair. However, it takes several applications and a good deal of time to produce the desired effect. The advantage of chamomile over chemical bleach is that it never gives a brassy or yellow tone.

To make a chamomile rinse to use after each shampoo, place 30 ml/2 tbsp dried chamomile flowers in 600 ml/ 1 pint boiling water. Simmer for about 15 minutes, strain and cool before use.

For a stronger rinse, add 125 g/1 cup dried chamomile flowers to 300 ml/ ½ pint boiling water and leave to steep for 15 minutes. Cool, simmer, and strain. Add the juice of a lemon plus 30 ml/ 2 tbsp rich cream conditioner. Comb through the hair and leave to dry – in the sun, if possible. Finally, shampoo and condition your hair as usual.

Choosing a New Colour

When choosing a colour a basic rule is to keep to one or two shades at each side of your original tone. It is best to try a temporary colourant first; if you like the result you can choose a semi-permanent or permanent colourant next time. If you want to be a platinum blonde and you are a natural brunette, you should seek the advice of a professional hairdresser.

There are two points to remember when considering a colour change. First, only have a colour change if your hair is in good condition; dry, porous hair absorbs colour too rapidly, leading to a patchy result. Second, your make-up may need changing to suit your new colour.

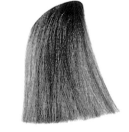

Special Techniques

Hairdressers over the years have devised colouring methods and techniques to create different effects. These are some of the choices available.

Flying colours

A combination of colours is applied with combs and brushes to the middle lengths and tips of the hair.

Highlights/lowlights

Fine strands of hair are tinted or bleached lighter or darker, or colour is added to give varying colour tones throughout the hair and to give the appearance of depth and texture. This technique can be called frosting or shimmering, particularly when bleach is used to give an overall lighter effect.

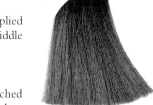

Slices

In this technique assorted colours are applied throughout the hair to emphasize the cut and to show movement.

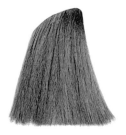

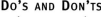

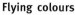

COVERING WHITE HAIR

To cover a few white hairs, use a temporary or semi-permanent colour that will last for six to eight weeks. Choose one that is similar to your natural colour. If the hair is brown, applying a warm brown colour will pick out the white areas and give lighter chestnut highlights. Alternatively, henna will give a glossy finish and produce stunning red highlights. For salt and pepper hair – hair with a mixed amount of white with the natural colour – try a longer lasting semi-permanent colour. These last for up to 20 shampoos and will also add shine.

When hair is completely white it can be covered with a permanent tint, but it will be necessary to update the colour every four to six weeks. You can enhance your natural shade of white by using toning shampoos, conditioners and styling products to remove brassiness and add some beautiful silvery tones.

CARING FOR COLOURED HAIR

Chlorinated and salt water, perspiration and the weather can all fade coloured hair, particularly hair that has been coloured red. Specialist products are available to help counteract fading, such as those with ultraviolet filters to protect coloured hair from the damaging effects of the sun's rays. Always rinse your hair thoroughly in chlorine-free water after swimming and use a shampoo designed for coloured hair, followed by a separate conditioner. Gently blot the hair after shampooing – never rub it vigorously as this ruffles the cuticle and can result in colour "escaping". It is a good idea to use an intensive conditioning treatment at least once a month to help prolong the colourant.

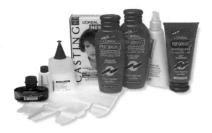

Above: Specially formulated care products.

BLEACHING

Bleaching gives a change in hair colour by removing colour from the hair. There are several different types of bleach available, ranging from mild brighteners that lift hair colour a couple of shades to more powerful mixes that completely strip hair of its natural colour.

Bleaching is difficult to do and is best left to a professional hairdresser. If misused it can be harsh and drying on the hair. For best results make sure your hair is in optimum condition before bleaching, and regularly apply an intensive conditioner to your hair afterwards.

COLOUR CORRECTION

If you have coloured your hair and want to go back to your natural colour without waiting for the colour to grow out, consult a professional hairdresser. Hair that has been tinted darker than its normal shade will have to be colour-stripped with a bleach bath until the desired colour is achieved. Hair that has been bleached or highlighted will need to be re-pigmented and then tinted to match the original colour. For best results, these processes should be carried out in a salon, using specialist products.

HELPFUL HINTS FOR HOME HAIR COLOURING

■ Always read the directions supplied with the product before you start, and follow them precisely. Make sure you first do a strand and skin sensitivity test.

■ If retouching the roots of tinted or bleached hair, apply new colour only to the regrowth area. Any overlap will result in uneven colour and porosity, which will affect the condition of your hair.

■ Don't colour your hair at home if the hair is split or visibly damaged, or if you have used bleach or henna; always allow previously treated hair to grow out first.

■ Avoid colouring your hair if taking prescribed drugs, as the chemical balance of your hair can alter. Check with your family doctor first.

■ If your hair has been permed, consult a hairdresser before using a hair colourant. If you are in any doubt about using a colour, check with the manufacturer or consult a professional hair colourist.

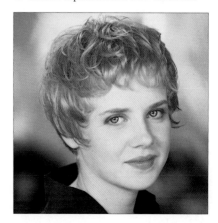

Above: A change of colour can give an instant lift to your hairstyle.

Permanent Solutions

Making straight hair curly is not a new idea. Women in ancient Egypt coated their hair in mud, wound it around wooden rods and then used the heat from the sun to create the curls. Waves that won't wash out are a more recent innovation. Improved formulations and sophisticated techniques have made perms the most versatile styling option in hairdressing.

HOW THEY WORK

Perms work by breaking down the inner structures (links) in your hair and reforming them to give a new shape. A perming lotion alters the keratin and breaks down the sulphur bonds that link the fibre-like cells together in the inner layers of the hair. When the fibres are loose, the hair is stretched over a curler or a perming rod to give a new shape.

Once the curlers or rods are in place, more lotion is applied and the perm is left to fix the new shape. The development time varies according to the condition and texture of the hair. When the development is complete, the changed links in the hair are re-formed into their new shape by the application of a neutralizer. The neutralizer contains an oxidizing agent that is responsible for closing up the broken links and producing the wave or curl – permanently.

The type of curl that is produced depends on the size of the curler. Generally speaking, the smaller the curler the smaller and tighter the curl, whereas medium to large curlers tend to give a much looser effect. The strength of the lotion and the type and texture of the hair can also make a difference.

HOME VERSUS SALON

Perming is a delicate operation, and it is often a good idea to leave it to trained and experienced professional hairdressers. The advantages of having hair permed in a salon are several. The hair is first analyzed to see whether it is in fit condition to take a perm; coloured, out-of-condition or over-processed hair may not be suitable and you will be then given specific advice on how to get your hair back into shape. A professional perm also offers more choice in the type of curl available – different strengths of lotion and different winding techniques all give a wider range of curls, many of which are not available in home perms.

Post Perm Tips

- Don't wash newly permed hair for 48 hours after processing as any stress can cause curls to relax.
- Use shampoos and conditioners formulated for permed hair to help retain the correct moisture balance and prolong the perm.
- Always use a wide-toothed comb and work from the ends upwards. Never brush the hair.
- Blot wet hair dry before styling to prevent stretching.
- Avoid using too much heat on permed hair. If possible, wash, condition and let dry naturally.
- If your perm has lost its bounce, mist with water or try a curl reviver. These are designed to put instant volume and bounce into permed hair.

DON'T DO IT YOURSELF IF . . .

- Your hair is very dry or damaged.
- You have bleached or highlighted your hair: it may be too fragile. If in doubt, check with your hairdresser.
- The traces of an old perm still remain in your hair.
- You suffer from a scalp disorder such as eczema or have broken, irritated skin.

Below: Spiral perming gives a ringlet effect on long hair.

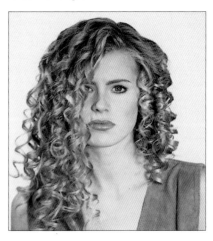

SALON PERMS – THE CHOICES

Professional hairdressers usually offer a number of different types of perm that are not available for home use.

Acid perms

These produce highly conditioned, flexible curls. They are ideally suited to hair that is fine, sensitive, fragile, damaged, or tinted, as they have a mildly acidic action that minimizes the risk of hair damage.

Alkaline perms

Alkaline perms give strong, firm curl results on normal and resistant hair.

Exothermic perms

These give bouncy, resilient curls. "Exothermic" refers to the gentle heat that is produced by the chemical reaction that occurs when the lotion is mixed. The heat allows the lotion to penetrate the hair cuticle, strengthening the hair as the hair moulds into its new shape.

PERMING TECHNIQUES

Any of the above types of perm can be used with different techniques to produce a number of results.

Body perms

These are soft, loose perms created by using large curlers, or sometimes rollers. The result is added volume with a hint of wave and movement rather than curls.

Root perms

To add lift and volume in the root area only. They are ideal for fine or short hair that tends to go flat.

Pin curl perms

These give soft, natural waves and curls, which are achieved by perming small sections of hair that have been pinned into pre-formed curls.

Stack perms

A stack perm gives curl and volume to one-length haircuts by means of different sized curlers. The hair on top of the head is left unpermed while the middle and ends have more curl and movement. The hair should be cut before the perm is applied.

Spiral perms

These create spiral curls by winding the hair around special curlers. The mass of curls makes long hair look much thicker.

Spot perms

Spot perms give support only on the area to which they are applied. If the hair needs lift the perm is applied just on the crown. They can also be used on the fringe (bangs) or on areas around the face.

Weave perms

Sections of hair are permed while the rest of the hair is left straight to give a mixture of texture and natural looking body and bounce, particularly on areas around the face.

REGROWTH PROBLEM

When a perm is growing out, the areas of new growth should only be permed if a barrier is created between old and new growth. The barrier can be a special cream or a plastic protector, both of which effectively prevent the perming lotion and neutralizer from touching previously permed areas.

Specially formulated products for re-perming a length of hair without damaging its structure are available from professional salons.

Below: Give thick hair a volume perm to produce a beautiful abundance of curls and the fullest look possible.

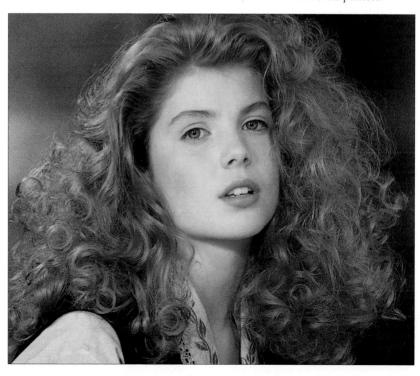

A Style to Suit your Face

Make the most of your looks by choosing a style that maximizes your best features. The first feature you should consider is your face shape – is it round, oval, square or long? If you are not sure what shape it is scrape your hair back off your face. Stand squarely in front of a mirror and use a lipstick to trace the outline of your face on to the mirror. When you stand back you should be able to see into which of the following categories your face shape falls.

THE SQUARE FACE

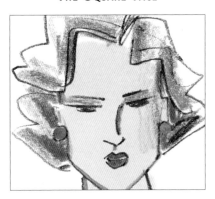

The square face is angular with a broad forehead and a square jawline. To make the best of this shape, choose a hairstyle with long layers, preferably one with soft waves or curls, as these create a softness that detracts from the hard lines. Part the hair on the side of the head and comb the fringe away from the face.
Styles to avoid: Severe geometric cuts – they will only emphasize squareness; long bobs with heavy fringes; severe styles in which the hair is scraped off the face and parted down the centre.

THE ROUND FACE

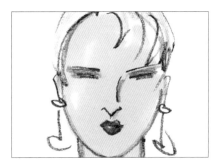

On the round face the distance between the forehead and the chin is about equal to the distance between the cheeks. Choose a style with a short fringe, which lengthens the face, and a short cut, which makes the face look thinner.
Styles to avoid: Curly styles, because they emphasize the roundness; very full, long hair or severe styles.

THE OVAL FACE

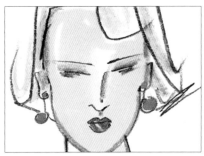

The oval face has wide cheekbones that taper down into a small chin and up to a narrow forehead. This is regarded as the perfect face shape and has the advantage of being able to wear any hairstyle well.

THE LONG FACE

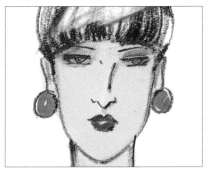

The long face has a high forehead and long chin and needs to be given the illusion of width. Soften the effect with short layers, or go for a bob with a fringe, to create horizontal lines. Curly or scrunch-dried bobs balance out a long face very well.
Styles to avoid: Styles without fringes, and long, straight, one-length cuts.

The Complete You

A hairstyle affects your whole appearance, not just that of your face. When choosing a new hairstyle you should take into account your overall body shape. If you are a traditional pear-shape don't choose an elfin hairstyle; it will draw attention to the lower half of your body, making your hips look wide. Petite women should avoid masses of very curly hair as this makes the head appear out of proportion with the rest of the body.

If You Wear Glasses . . .

Try to choose frames and
a hairstyle that complement each
other. Large spectacles could spoil
a neat, feathery cut, and very fine
frames could be overpowered by
a large, voluminous style. Remember
to take your glasses to the salon
when having your hair restyled
so that your stylist can take their
shape into consideration when
deciding on the overall effect.

SPECIFIC PROBLEMS

■ Prominent nose: choose a hairstyle
that incorporates softness into your
appearance. A wispy fringe would work
well, and a light perm would add height
and movement, to balance out your face.

■ Pointed chin: you need to style your
hair with plenty of width at the jawline.
Don't have your hair cut too short.

■ Low forehead: choose a style with
a wispy fringe, rather than one with
a full fringe. Choose softer styles and
avoid anything too severe.

■ High forehead: this is best disguised
with a mid-length fringe.

■ Receding chin: select a hairstyle that
comes just below chin level, ideally
with lots of waves or curls around
your shoulders.

■ Uneven hairline: a fringe should
easily manage to conceal this problem.

Right: Your hairstyle has a big influence
on your appearance, so be honest with
yourself and take a critical look in the
mirror before choosing a new style.

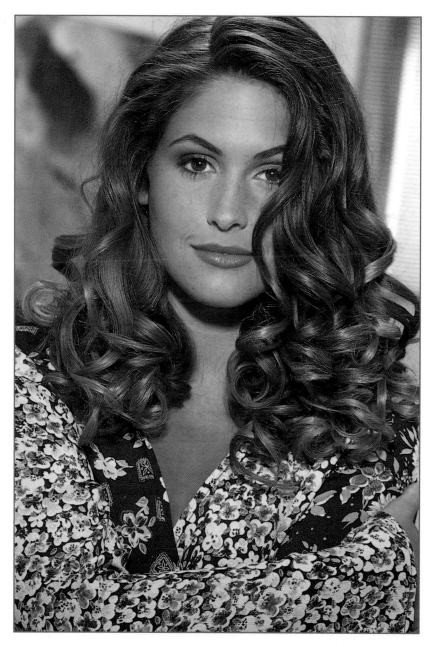

Styling Tools

The right tools not only make hairstyling more fun, but also make it much easier. Brushes, combs and pins are the basic tools of styling. The following is a guide to help you choose what is most suitable from the wide range that is available.

BRUSHES

Brushes are made of bristles, which may be natural hog bristle, plastic, nylon or wire. The bristles are embedded in a wooden, plastic or moulded rubber base and set in tufts or rows. This allows loose hair to collect in the grooves without interfering with the action of the bristles. The spacing of the tufts plays an important role – generally, the wider the spacing between the rows the easier the brush will flow through the hair.

The role of brushing

Brushes help to remove tangles and knots and smooth the hair. The action of brushing from the roots to the ends removes dead skin cells and dirt and encourages the cuticles to lie flat, reflecting the light. Brushing also stimulates the circulation, promoting hair growth.

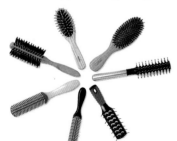

Above: Brushes should be carefully chosen and well looked after.

Tip

Replace brushes and combs with damaged bristles or broken teeth; the sharp edges can damage your scalp. Keep your brushes and combs to yourself, never lend to other people.

Cleaning

All brushes should be cleaned, at least once a week, by pulling out dead hairs and washing in warm, soapy water, then rinsing thoroughly. Natural bristle brushes should be left to dry naturally. If you use a pneumatic brush with a rubber cushion base, block the air hole with a matchstick before washing.

Plastic, nylon or wire bristles

All of these bristles are easily cleaned and are heat resistant, so they are good for blow-drying. They are available in a variety of shapes and styles. Cushioned brushes give good flexibility as they glide through the hair, preventing tugging and helping to remove knots. They are also non-static. A major disadvantage is that the ends can be harsh, so try to choose bristles with rounded or ball tips.

TYPES OF BRUSH

Circular or radial brushes

These brushes come in a variety of sizes and are circular or semicircular in shape. Circular or radial brushes have either mixed bristles for finishing a style, a rubber pad with nylon bristles for general use or metal pins specifically for styling. They are used to control naturally curly, permed and wavy hair and are ideal for blow-drying.

Flat or half-round brushes

These are ideal for wet or dry hairstyling and blow-drying. Normally they are made of nylon bristles in a rubber base.

Pneumatic brushes

These brushes have a domed rubber base with bristles set in tufts. They can be plastic, natural bristle or both.

Vent brushes

Vent brushes have hollow centres and special bristle, or pin, patterns that are designed to lift and disentangle hair. The air circulates freely through both the brush and the hair so the hair dries faster.

COMBS

Good quality combs have saw-cut teeth: each individual tooth is cut into the comb, so there are no sharp edges. Avoid cheap plastic combs that are made in a mould and form lines down the centre of the teeth. These scrape away the cuticle layers of the hair, eventually causing damage. Use a wide-toothed comb for disentangling and combing conditioner through the hair. Fine tail combs are for styling; Afro combs are for curly hair; and styling combs are for grooming.

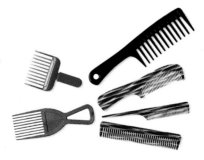

Above: Your choice of comb will vary according to the texture of your hair.

PINS AND CLIPS

These are indispensable for sectioning and securing hair during setting and for putting hair up. Most pins are available with untipped, plain ends, or cushion tipped ends. Non-reflective finishes are available, so the pins are less noticeable in the hair, and most are made of metal, plastic or stainless steel. Colours and styles vary from plain to adorned and highly decorative fashion accessories.

Double-pronged clips

These are most frequently used for making pin or barrel curls. Grips on the clips give added security to all types of curls, French pleats and the most intricately upswept styles.

Heavy hairpins

These are made of strong metal and come either waved or straight. They are ideal for securing rollers or for putting hair up.

Fine hairpins

These are used for dressing hair. They are delicate and prone to bend out of shape, so they should only be used to secure small amounts of hair. Fine hairpins are easily concealed, especially if you use a matching colour. They are sometimes used to secure pin curls during setting as heavier clips can leave a mark.

Sectioning clips

These clips have a single prong. They are often used to hold hair while working on another section, or securing pin curls.

Twisted pins

These are fashioned like a screw and are used to secure hairstyles such as chignons and French pleats.

ROLLERS

Rollers vary in diameter, length and the material from which they are made. Smooth rollers – those without spikes or brushes – will give the sleekest finish, but can be difficult to put in. More popular are brush rollers, especially the self-fixing variety that do not need pins or clips.

> **Tip**
> The smaller the roller, the tighter the curl. Keep the tension even when winding and do not buckle the ends of the hair.

SHAPERS

Shapers were inspired by the principle of rag-rolling hair and are a natural way to curl hair. Soft "twist tie" shapers are made from pliable rubber, plastic or cotton, with a tempered wire in the centre to enable it to bend into shape. The waves or curls that are produced are soft and bouncy and the technique is gentle enough for permed or tinted hair.

To use, section clean, dry hair and pull to a firm tension, "trapping" the end in a shaper that you have previously doubled over. Roll down to the roots and fold over to secure. Leave for 30–60 minutes without heat. For a more voluminous style, twist the hair before curling.

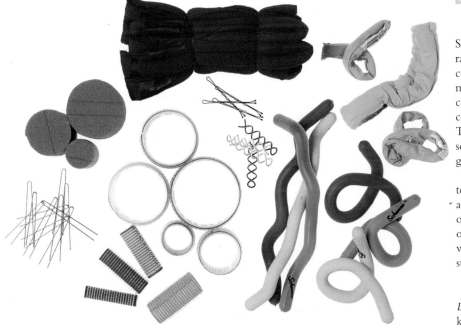

Left: Pin, clip, grip, roll, curl or tie – keep a supply of "extras" to hand for styling your hair.

Style Easy

The combination of practice and the right styling products enables you to achieve a salon finish at home. The products listed below will enable you to do it in style.

GELS

Gels come in varying degrees of viscosity, from a thick jelly to a liquid spray. They are sometimes called sculpting lotions and are used for precise styling. Use them to lift roots, tame wisps, create tendrils, calm static, heat set and give structure to curls. Wet gels can be used for sculpting styles.

HAIRSPRAY

Traditionally, hairspray was used to hold a style in place; today varying degrees of stiffness are available to suit all needs. Use hairspray to keep the hair in place, get curl definition when scrunching and mist over rollers when setting.

MOUSSE

Mousse is the most versatile styling product. It comes as a foam and can be used on wet or dry hair. Mousses contain conditioning agents and proteins to nurture and protect the hair. They are available in different strengths, designed to give soft to maximum holding power, and can be used to lift flat roots or smooth frizz. Use when blow-drying, scrunching and diffuser-drying.

SERUMS

Serums, glossers, polishes and shine sprays are made from oils or silicones, which improve shine and softness by forming a microscopic film on the surface of the hair. Formulations vary from light and silky to heavier ones with an oily feel. They smooth the cuticle, encouraging the tiny scales to lie flat and reflect the light, making the hair shine. Use to improve the feel of the hair, to combat static, de-frizz, add shine and gloss and to temporarily repair split ends.

STYLING OR SETTING LOTIONS

Styling lotions contain resins that form a film on the hair and aid setting and protect the hair from heat damage. There are formulations for dry, coloured or sensitized hair; others give volume and shine. Use for roller-setting, scrunching, blow-drying and natural drying.

> **Tip**
> If you are using a styling lotion for heat setting, look for formulations that offer thermal protection.

WAXES, POMADES AND CREAMS

These products are made from natural waxes, softened with other ingredients such as mineral oils and lanolin to make them pliable. Some pomades contain vegetable wax and oil to give gloss and sheen. Other formulations produce foam and are water soluble, and leave no residue. Use these products for controlling frizz and static.

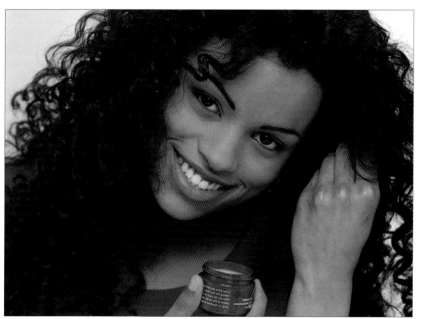

Above: Rub a little wax between the palms of your hands, then work into the curls with the fingertips to give separation and shine to thick, curly hair.

Appliances

Heated styling appliances allow you to style your hair quickly, efficiently and easily. A wide range of heated appliances is available.

AIR STYLERS

Air stylers combine the versatility of a hairdryer with the convenience of a styling wand. They operate on the same principle as a hairdryer, blowing warm air through the styler. Many come with a variety of clip-on options, including brushes, prongs and tongs. Use for creating waves and volume at the roots.

CRIMPERS

Crimpers consist of two ridged metal plates that produce uniform patterned crimps in straight lines in the hair. The hair must be straightened first, either by blow-drying or using flat irons. The crimper is then used to give waves or ripples. Use for special styling effects or to increase volume.

HAIRDRYERS

Choose a dryer that has a range of heat and speed settings so that the hair can be power-dried on high heat, finished on a lower heat, and then used with cool air to set the style. The life expectancy of a hairdryer averages between 200–300 hours. Use for blow-drying.

DIFFUSERS AND NOZZLES

Originally, diffusers were intended for drying curly hair, encouraging curl formation by spreading the airflow over the hair so the curls are not literally blown away. The prongs on the diffuser head also help to increase volume at the roots and give lift. Diffusers with flat heads are designed for gentle drying without ruffling and are more suitable for shorter styles. The newest type of diffuser has long, straight prongs that are designed to inject volume into straight hair while giving a smooth finish.

HEATED ROLLERS

A set of heated rollers will normally comprise a selection of 20 small, medium and large rollers, with colour-coded clips to match. Early models came with spikes, but newer developments include ribbed rubber surfaces, designed to be kinder to the hair.

The speed at which the rollers heat up varies, depending on the type of roller, but all rollers cool down completely in 30 minutes. Use heated rollers for quick sets, to give curl and body. They are ideal for preparing hair for dressing into styles.

> **Tip**
> Heat drying encourages static, causing hair to fly away. Reduce static by lightly touching your hair, or mist your hair brush with hairspray to calm the hair.

Below: Rollers make great styling tools.

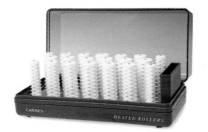

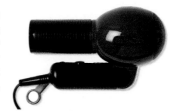

Above: Hairdryers are an essential piece of equipment for quick-drying and styling hair.

STRAIGHTENERS

Straighteners are similar to crimpers but have flat plates to iron out frizz or curl. Use for "pressing" really curly hair.

TONGS

Tongs consist of a barrel, or prong, and a depressor groove. The thickness of the barrel varies, and the size of the tong that is used depends on whether small, medium or large curls are required.

HOT BRUSHES

Hot brushes are easier to handle than tongs and come in varying sizes for creating curls of different sizes. Wind down the lengths of the hair, hold for a few seconds until the heat has penetrated through the hair, then gently remove. Cordless hot brushes use gas cartridges or batteries to produce heat and are used to give root lift, curl and movement.

TRAVEL DRYERS

Travel dryers are ideal for taking on holiday. They are usually miniature versions of standard dryers, and some are even available with their own small diffusers. Check that the dryer you buy has dual voltage and a travel case.

Blow-drying

ollow our step-by-step sequence for the smoothest, sleekest blow-dried hairstyle ever.

Styling Checklist
You will need:
styling comb
hairdryer
mousse
clip
styling brush
serum

1 Shampoo and condition your hair, as usual. Comb through gently with a wide-toothed comb to remove any tangles.

2 Partially dry your hair to remove excess moisture. Apply a handful of mousse to the palm of your hand. Using your other hand, spread the mousse through the hair, distributing it evenly from the tips to the ends.

3 Divide your hair into two sections by clipping the top and sides out of the way. Then, working on the hair that is left free and taking one small section at a time, hold the dryer in one hand and a styling brush in the other. Place the brush underneath the first section of hair, positioning it at the roots. Keeping the tension on the hair taut, move the brush towards the end, directing the air flow from the dryer so that it follows the downwards movement of the brush.

4 Curve the brush under at the ends to achieve a slight bend. Concentrate on drying the root area first, repeatedly introducing the brush to the roots once it has moved down the length of the hair. Continue the movement until the first section of the hair is dry. Repeat step 4 until the whole of the back section is dry.

5 Release a section of hair from the top and dry it in the same manner. Continue in this way until you have dried all your hair. Finish by smoothing a few drops of serum through the hair to flatten any flyaway ends.

Tips
■ Use the highest heat setting to remove excess moisture, then switch to medium to finish drying.
■ Point the air flow downwards. This smoothes the cuticles and makes the hair shine.
■ Make sure each section is dry before going on to the next.

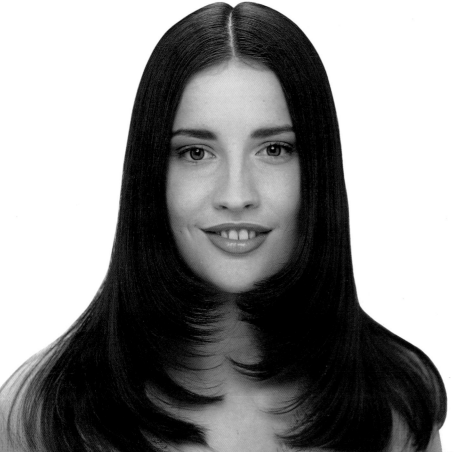

Roll-Up

Roller sets form the basis of many hairstyles; use them to smooth hair, add waves or soft curls, or to provide a foundation for an upswept style.

Styling Checklist
You will need:
styling lotion
tail comb
self-fixing rollers or brush
rollers and pins
hand or hood dryer (optional)
hairspray

1 Shampoo and condition your hair, then partially dry to remove excess moisture. Mist with a styling lotion.

2 For a basic set, take a 5 cm/2 in section of hair (or a section the same width as your roller) from the centre front and comb it straight up, smoothing out any tangles. Wrap the ends of the sectioned hair around the roller, taking care not to buckle the hair. Then wind the roller down firmly, towards the scalp, keeping the tension even and comfortably taut.

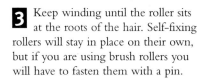

3 Keep winding until the roller sits at the roots of the hair. Self-fixing rollers will stay in place on their own, but if you are using brush rollers you will have to fasten them with a pin.

4 Continue around the whole head, always taking the same width of hair. Re-mist the hair with styling lotion if it begins to dry out.

5 Leave the finished set to dry naturally, or dry it with a diffuser attachment on your hand dryer, or with a hood dryer. If using artificial heat sources let the dry hair cool before you remove the rollers. Brush through the hair following the direction of the set. Mist the brush with hairspray and use to smooth any stray hairs.

Tips
■ Use large diameter rollers for sleek, wavy looks, smaller rollers for curlier styles.
■ Always use sections of equal width when setting your hair or you will get an uneven result.
■ For maximum volume and control, let the hair cool down completely before brushing through.
■ A bristle brush will give a smoother finish to the style.
■ If the finished set is too curly after brushing through, loosen the curl with a brush used with a hand dryer.
■ To create extra volume and height use a fine-toothed comb to backcomb the roots.

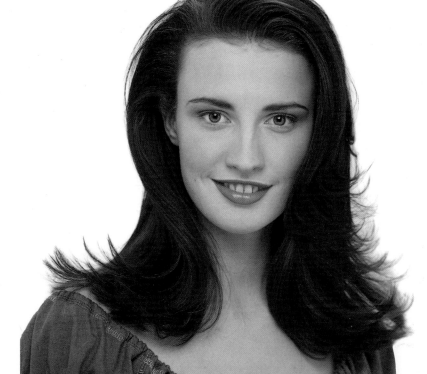

Finger-drying

This is a quick method of drying and styling your hair. It relies on the heat released from your hands rather than the heat from a dryer. Finger-drying is suitable for short to mid-length hair.

Styling Checklist
You will need:
spray gel
styling comb

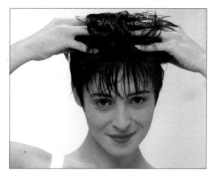

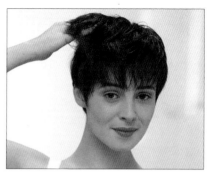

1 Shampoo and condition your hair as usual, then spray with gel and comb through gently.

2 Run your fingers upwards and forwards, from the roots to the ends.

3 Lift the hair at the crown to get height at the roots.

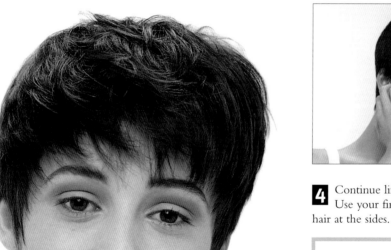

4 Continue lifting as the hair dries. Use your fingertips to flatten the hair at the sides.

Tip
Finger-drying is the best way to dry damaged hair or to encourage waves in naturally curly, short hair.

Barrel Curls

One of the simplest sets is achieved by curling the hair around the fingers and then pinning the curl in place. Barrel curls create a soft set.

1 Shampoo and condition your hair; apply setting lotion and comb through from the roots to the ends. Take a small section of hair (about 2.5 cm/1 in) and smooth it upwards.

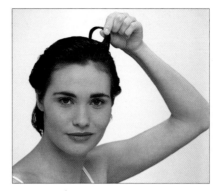

2 Loop the hair into a large curl.

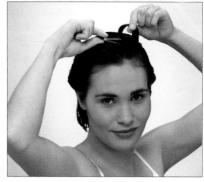

3 Clip the curl in place.

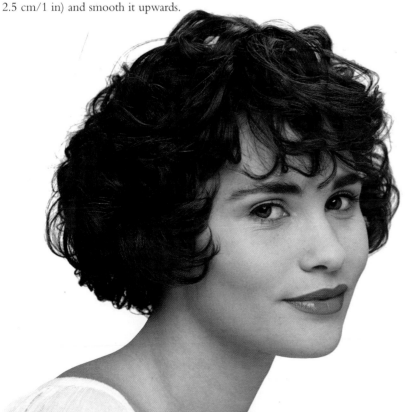

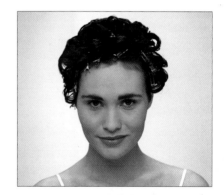

4 Continue to curl the rest of the hair in the same way.

5 Dry the hair with a hood dryer or allow it to dry naturally. Remove the clips. To achieve a tousled look rake your fingers through your hair. For a smoother finish use a hair brush.

Soft-setting

Fabric rollers are the modern version of old-fashioned rags. Apart from being very easy to use they are kind to the hair and give a highly effective set.

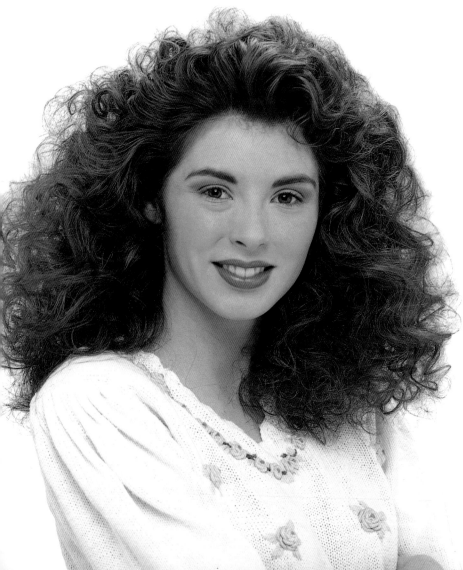

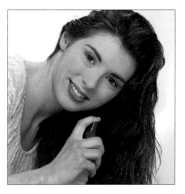

1 Dampen the hair with styling lotion, making sure you distribute it evenly from the roots to the ends.

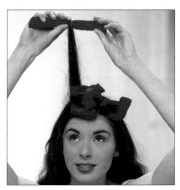

2 Using sections of hair about 2.5 cm/1 in wide, curl the end of the hair around a fabric roller and wind the roller down towards the scalp, taking care not to buckle the ends of the hair.

Tip
For even more volume, twist each section of hair lengthwise before winding it on to the fabric roller.

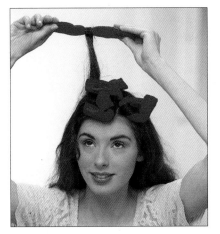

3 Continue winding the roller right down to the roots.

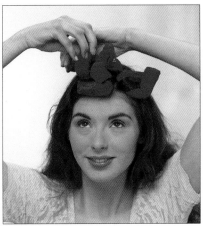

4 To fasten, simply bend each end of the fabric roller towards the centre. This grips the hair and holds it in place.

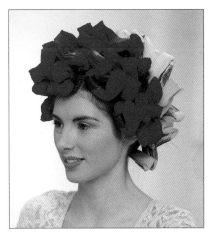

5 Leave to dry naturally when the complete set of rollers is in place.

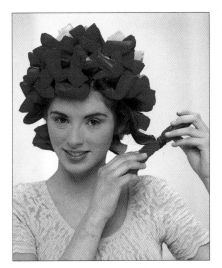

6 When the hair is dry, remove the rollers by unbending the ends and unwinding the hair.

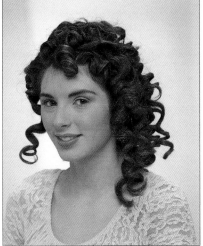

7 When all the rollers have been removed the hair falls into firm corkscrew curls.

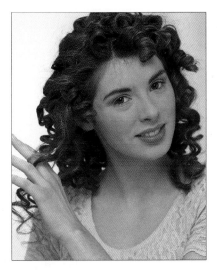

8 Working on one curl at a time, rake your fingers through the hair, teasing out each curl. The result will be a full, voluminous finish.

Tong and Twist

Tongs can be used to smooth the hair and add just the right amount of movement.

1 Shampoo, condition and dry your hair. Apply a mist of styling lotion. Never use mousse as it will stick to the tongs and bake into the hair. Divide off a small section of hair.

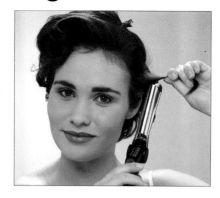

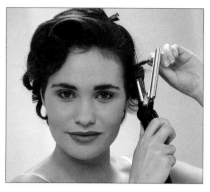

2 Press the depressor to open the tongs.

3 Wind the section of hair around the barrel of the tongs.

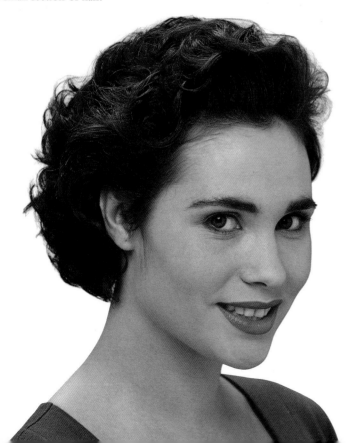

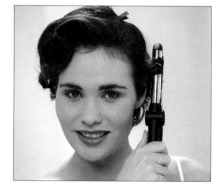

4 Release the depressor to hold the hair in place and wait a few seconds for the curl to form. Remove the tongs and leave the hair to cool while you work on the rest of your hair. Style by raking through with your fingers.

Tip
Never use tongs on bleached hair. The high heat can damage the hair, causing brittleness and breakage.

Airwaves

Air styling makes use of gentle heat and combines it with the moisture in your hair to give a long lasting curl.

1 Shampoo and condition your hair. Mist with styling lotion.

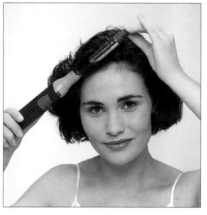

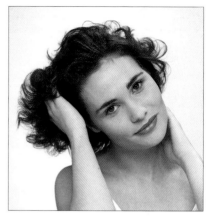

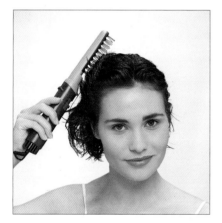

3 Clip on the tong attachment and continue shaping the hair by wrapping it around the tongs.

4 Repeat steps 2 and 3 until the whole head is curled and waved. When the hair is completely dry rake your fingers through it.

2 Using the brush attachment on the styler, start drying the hair. Lift each section to allow the heat to dry the roots.

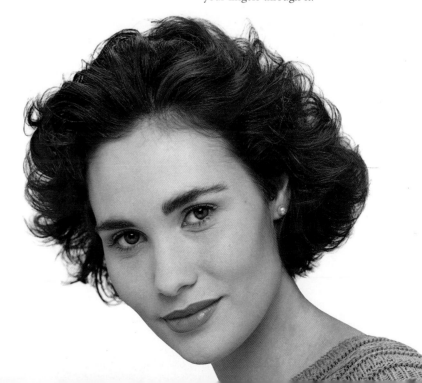

Dragged Side Braids

Curly hair can be controlled, yet still allowed to flow free, by braiding it at the sides and allowing the hair at the back to fall in a mass of curls.

Styling Checklist
Time: 5 minutes
Ease/Difficulty: Easy
Hair type: Long and naturally
curly or permed
You will need:
styling comb
covered bands
hair grips

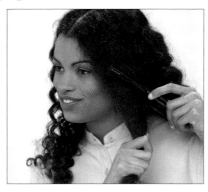

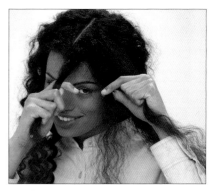

1 Part your hair in the centre and divide off a large section at the side, combing it as flat as possible to the head.

2 Divide the section into three equal strands and hold them apart.

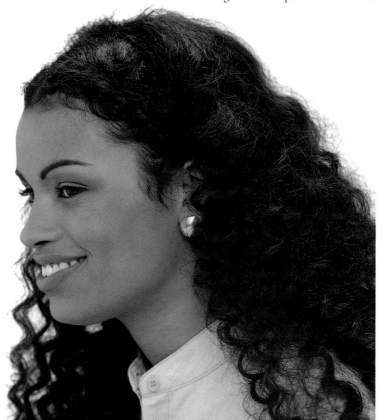

3 Make a dragged braid by pulling the strands of hair towards your face and then taking the right strand over the centre strand, the left strand over the centre, and the right over the centre again, keeping the braid in position.

4 Continue braiding to the end and secure the end with a covered band. Tuck the braid behind your ear and grip it in place, then make a second braid on the other side.

Ribbon Bow

A simple ponytail is given added interest by binding with ribbon and finishing with a bow.

Styling Checklist
Time: 5 minutes
Ease/difficulty: Easy
Hair type: Long and straight
You will need:
brush or styling comb
covered band
about 1 m/1 yd of ribbon

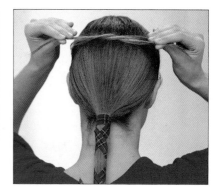

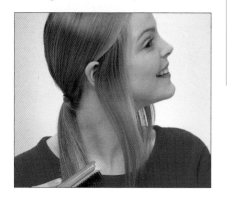

1 Brush or comb your hair smoothly back into a neat ponytail, leaving a small section free at either side. Secure the ponytail with a covered band.

3 Cross the ribbon over the ponytail, continuing until you are 5–7.5 cm/ 2–3 in from the end. Tie the ribbon into a bow. Smooth out the side sections of hair and tie them into a neat bow at the centre back of your head above the be-ribboned ponytail. Secure with a hairpin if necessary.

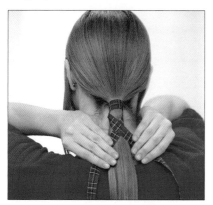

2 Position the centre of the ribbon over the band as shown, pulling the ends of the ribbon taut.

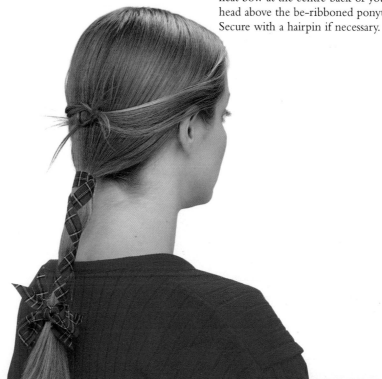

Ponytail Styler

Asimple ponytail can be transformed into something very sophisticated using this clever styler.

Tip

The same technique can be used on wet hair as long as you apply gel first, combing it through evenly before styling.

Styling Checklist

Time: 10–15 minutes, depending on experience
Ease/difficulty: Quite easy, but can be fiddly
Hair type: Long, straight, one length
You will need:
covered band
ponytail styler

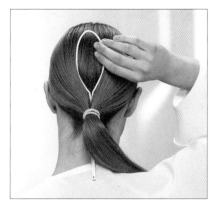

1 Clasp the hair into a neat ponytail and secure it with a covered band. Insert the styler as shown.

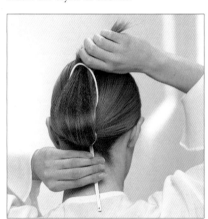

2 Pull the ponytail up and thread it through the styler.

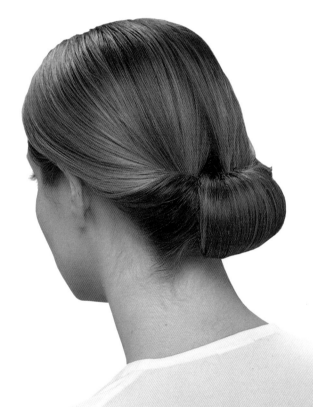

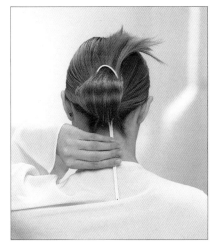
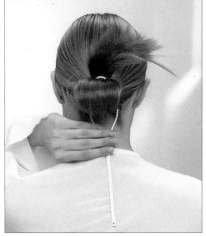
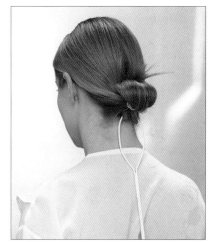

3 Begin to pull the styler down . . .

4 . . . continue pulling . . .

5 . . . so the ponytail pulls through . . .

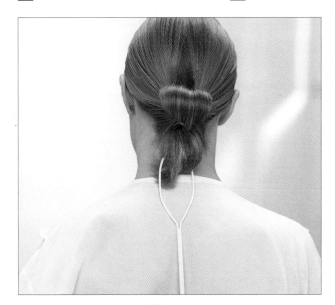
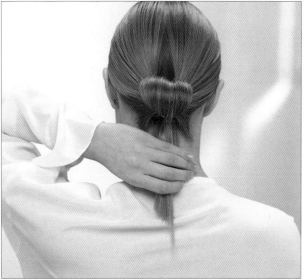

6 . . . and emerges underneath.

7 Smooth the hair with your hand and insert the styler again, repeating steps 2 to 6 once more to give a neat and smooth chignon loop.

Curly Styler

The ponytail styler can also be used to tame a mass of curls, creating a ponytail with a simple double twist.

Tip

When inserting the styler through a ponytail, carefully move it from side to side in order to create enough room to pull the looped end of the styler through more easily.

Styling Checklist

Time: 5 minutes
Ease/difficulty: Easy
Hair type: Long and naturally curly or permed.
You will need:
widely spaced tooth comb
covered band
ponytail styler
mousse

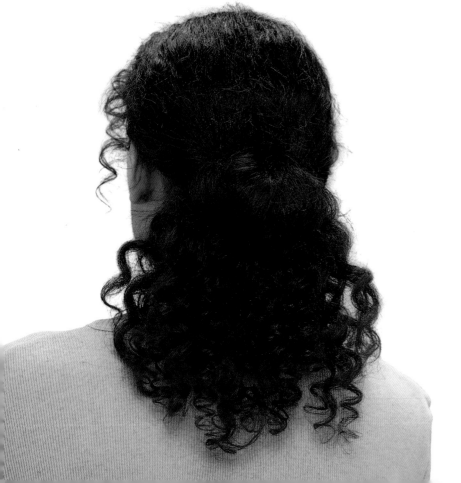

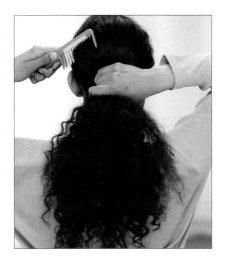

1 Use a comb with widely spaced teeth to smooth the hair back and into a ponytail. Secure with a covered hair band.

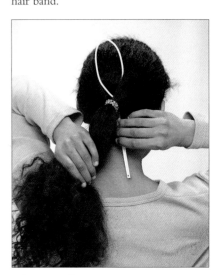

2 Insert the styler as shown.

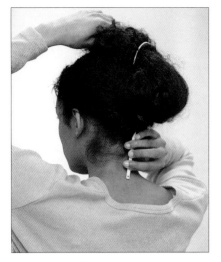

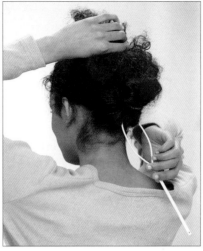

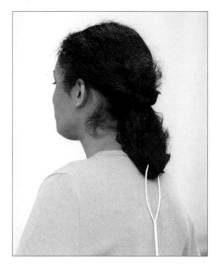

3 Pull the ponytail up and thread it through the styler.

4 Begin to pull the styler down . . .

5 . . . continue pulling . . .

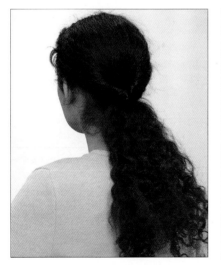

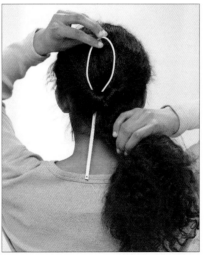

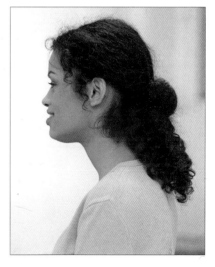

6 . . . so that the ponytail pulls all the way through.

7 Repeat steps 2 to 6.

8 Apply a little mousse to your hands and use it to re-form the curls, scrunching to achieve a good shape.

French Braid

This elegant, sophisticated braid looks complicated but it does get easier with practice.

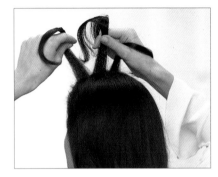

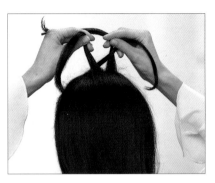

1 Take a section of hair from the front of the head and divide into three even strands. Braid once, taking the left and right strands over the centre strand.

2 Hold the braid and use your thumbs to gather additional hair (approximately 1 cm/½ in strips) from each side of the head. Add these to the original strands. Braid the strands once again.

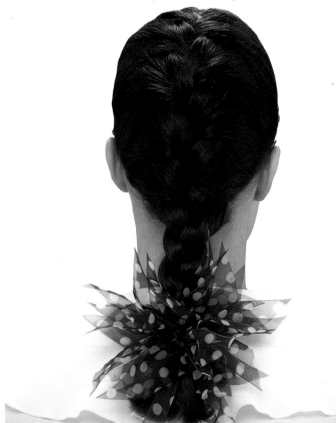

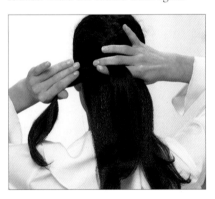

3 Continue in this way, picking up more hair as you continue down the braid. Secure the French braid with a covered band and add a scrunchie.

Tip
Shorter front layers can be woven into this type of braid, as when growing out a fringe, for example.

Double-stranded Braids

These clever braids have a fishbone pattern, which gives an unusual look.

Styling Checklist
Time: 10 minutes
Ease/difficulty: Needs practice
Hair type: Long and straight
You will need:
styling comb
covered bands
coloured feathers
two short lengths of fine leather

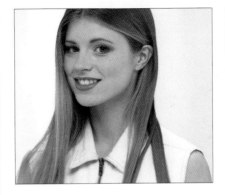

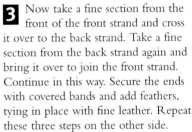

2 Divide the hair on one side of your head into two strands, then take a fine section from the back of the back strand and take it over to join the front strand, as shown.

3 Now take a fine section from the front of the front strand and cross it over to the back strand. Take a fine section from the back strand again and bring it over to join the front strand. Continue in this way. Secure the ends with covered bands and add feathers, tying in place with fine leather. Repeat these three steps on the other side.

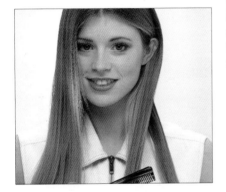

1 Part your hair in the centre and comb it straight.

Crown Braids

By braiding the crown hair and allowing the remaining hair to frame the face you can achieve an interesting contrast of textures.

Styling Checklist
Time: 15 minutes
Ease/difficulty: Needs practice
Hair type: Mid-length to long and naturally curly or permed
You will need:
large clip
styling comb
small covered bands
Alice headband

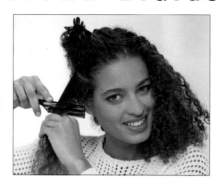

1 Clip up the top hair on one side of your head, leaving the back hair free. Take a small section of hair at ear level and comb it straight.

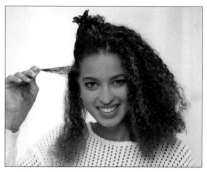

2 Start braiding quite tightly, doing one cross (right strand over centre, left over centre), and gradually bring more hair into the outside strands.

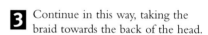

3 Continue in this way, taking the braid towards the back of the head.

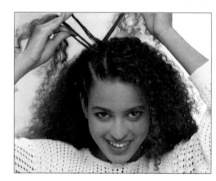

4 Make another parting about 2.5 cm/1 in parallel to and above the previous braid, and repeat the process. Continue in this way until all the front hair has been braided. Secure the braids with small covered bands and scrunch the remaining hair into large curls to increase the volume. Finally, add a decorative Alice band.

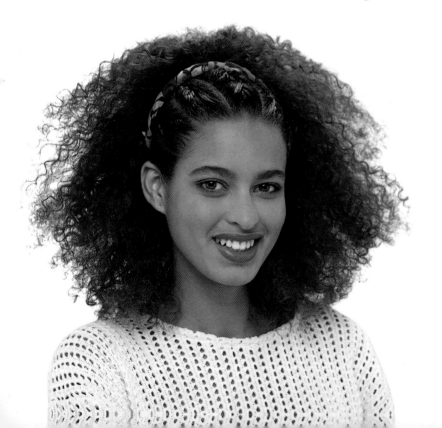

Rick-rack Braids

You can achieve a colourful look by braiding the hair with rick-rack to give a young, fresh style.

Styling Checklist
Time: Time consuming
Ease/difficulty: Quite easy
Hair type: Mid-length to long and naturally curly or permed
You will need:
coloured rick-rack (about 3.5 m/3.5 yd of three different colours)
hairpins and small covered bands

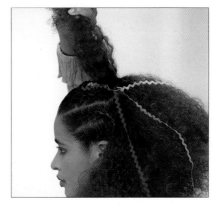

2 Take a section of hair and divide it into three strands, aligning one piece of rick-rack with each strand.

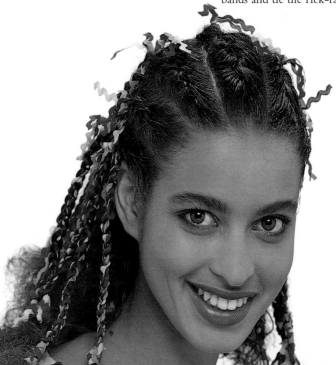

3 Begin braiding, taking the right strand over the centre strand, the left over the centre, right over the centre, and so on. Continue braiding down to the ends, add small covered bands and tie the rick-rack to fasten.

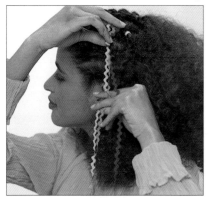

1 Braid the front of the hair. Tie three strands of rick-rack at one end and pin to the band of one braid.

Tip
Naturally curly or permed hair benefits from regular intensive conditioning treatments.

Basketweave Braid

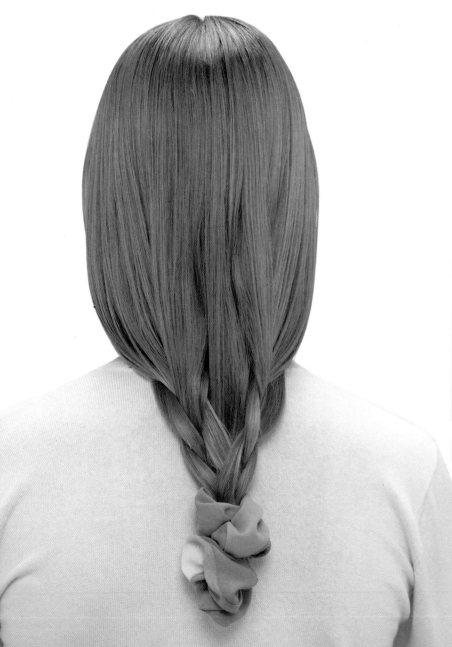

Enlist the help of a friend to help you create this unusual braid style.

Styling Checklist
Time: 10 minutes
Ease/difficulty: Needs practice
Hair type: Mid-length to long
You will need:
styling comb
scrunchie

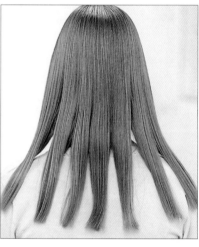

1 Divide the hair into seven equal strands – three strands on either side of the face and one at the centre back.

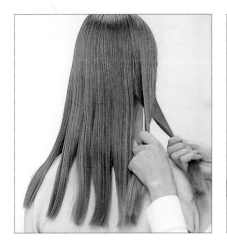

2 Starting at the right-hand side, cross the first strand (the strand nearest the face) over the second strand.

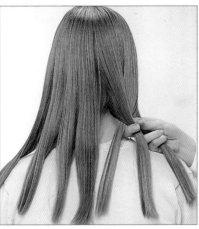

3 Cross the third strand over what is now the second strand, as shown.

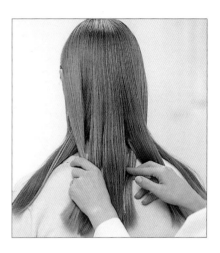

4 Repeat steps 2 and 3 on the left side. What was originally the first strand in each group will now be the third strand.

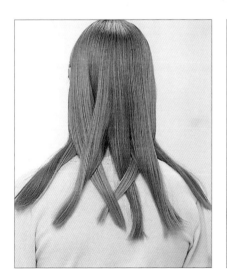

5 Take the third strand on the right-hand side over the central strand, and under the third strand on the left-hand side.

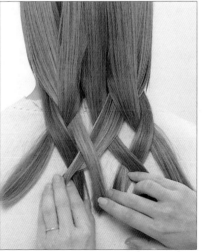

6 Now bring the first strand on the right-hand side over the second strand and under the central strand.

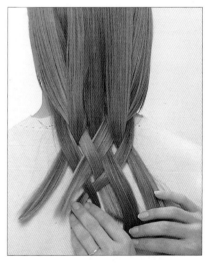

7 Repeat step 6 on the left side. Finally, clasp with a scrunchie to secure in place.

Twist and Coil

This style starts with a simple ponytail, is easy to do and looks stunning.

Styling Checklist
Time: 10 minutes
Ease/difficulty: Easy
Hair type: Long, one length,
straight hair
You will need:
small covered band
shine spray
hairpins
1 m/1 yd strip of sequins

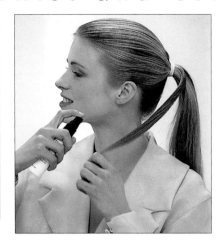

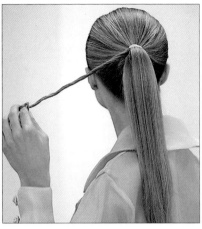

1 Brush the hair and smooth it back, securing it in a ponytail using a small covered band.

2 Divide off a section of hair and mist with shine spray for some gloss.

3 Holding the ends of a section, twist the hair until it rolls back on itself to form a coil.

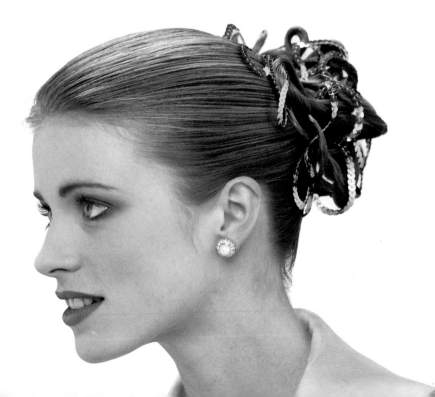

4 Position the coil in a loop as shown and secure in place using hairpins. Continue in this manner until all the hair has been coiled. Decorate by intertwining with a strip of sequins.

Cameo Braid

A classic bun is given extra panache by encircling it with a braid.

Styling Checklist
Time: 10 minutes
Ease/difficulty: Needs practice
Hair type: Long and straight
You will need:
small covered band
bun ring
hairpins

1 Smooth the hair into a ponytail, leaving one section of the hair free.

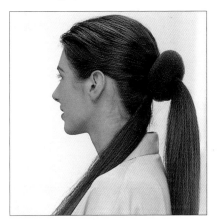

2 Place a bun ring over the ponytail.

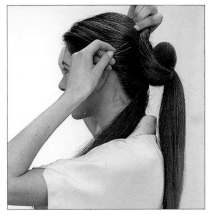

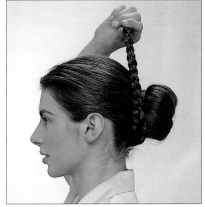

3 Take approximately one-third of the hair from the ponytail and wrap it around the bun ring, securing with pins. Repeat with the other two-thirds of the hair.

4 Braid the section of hair that was left out of the ponytail, right strand over centre strand, left over centre and so on, and wrap the braid around the base of the bun, then secure with pins.

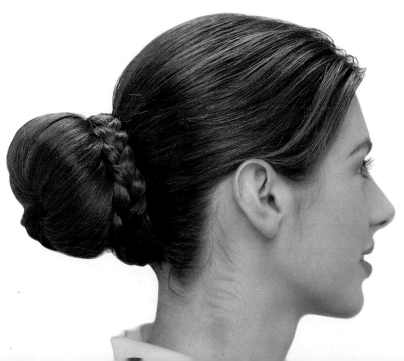

Rope Braid

A simple braid is entwined with rope to give an unusual finish.

Styling Checklist
Time: 10 minutes.
Ease/difficulty: Easy
Hair type: Long and straight
You will need:
styling comb
hair clip and hairpins
three equal lengths of rope,
tied at one end
small covered bands

1 Divide off the top section of hair and comb it through. Clip in place and pin the rope in place on the crown.

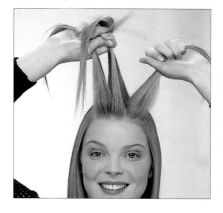

2 Separate the front piece of hair into three equal strands. Begin to braid.

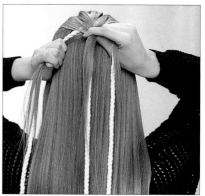

3 When the braid reaches the top of the rope, merge a strand of rope with each strand of braid and continue working down to the ends.

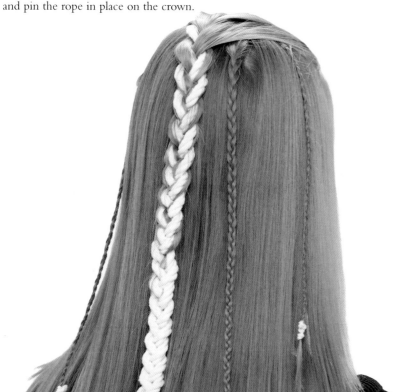

4 Secure with a covered band. Then make four more small braids, equally spaced around the head, and secure each end with covered bands.

City Slicker

Transform your hair in a matter of minutes into this punchy young style, using gel to slick it into shape.

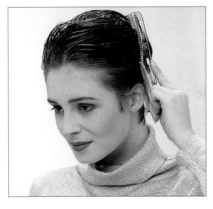

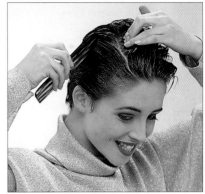

1 Take a generous amount of gel and apply it to the hair from the roots down to the ends.

3 Comb the hair into shape using a styling comb to give movement.

4 Shape the hair to form a quiff and sleek down the sides and back.

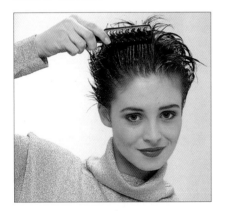

2 Use a vent brush, a comb or your fingers to distribute the gel evenly through the hair.

Tip
Make sure you distribute the gel evenly all over your hair before styling.

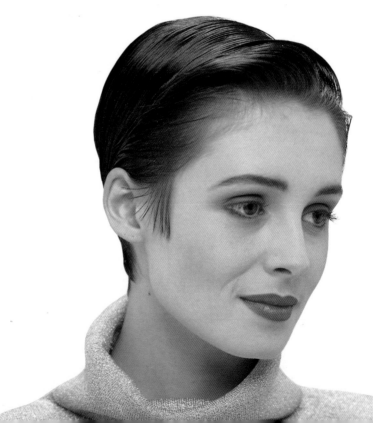

Mini Braids

This fresh and upbeat look is an ideal style for teenagers.

Styling Checklist

Time: Rather time consuming
Ease/difficulty: Needs practice
Hair type: Long and straight
You will need:
styling wax
small covered bands
a length of ribbon about 1 m/1 yd
long, cut into 6 pieces

Tip

To smooth any flyaway ends
rub a few drops of serum between
the palms of your hands and
smooth over the hair.

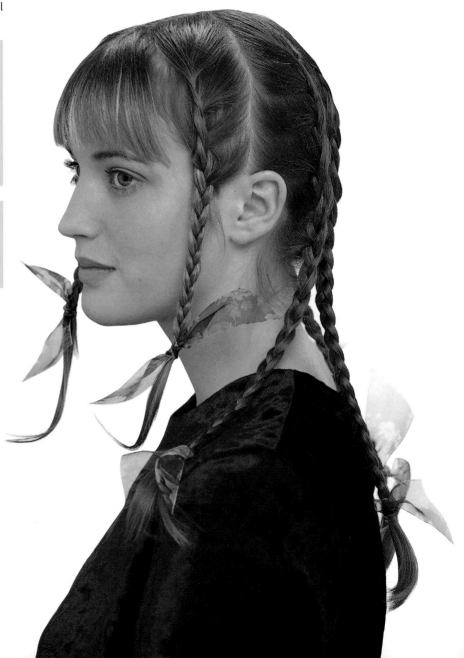

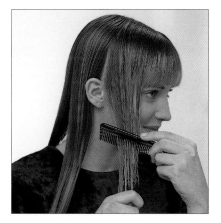

1 Part the hair in the centre and smooth with a little wax that has first been warmed between the palms of your hands before spreading over the hair.

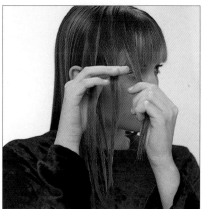

2 Divide off a section at one side, as shown, and divide again into three equal parts.

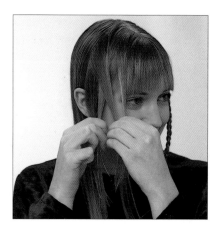

3 Braid the hair by placing the right strand over the centre strand, the left over the centre, right over the centre, and so on, pulling the braid slightly towards the face.

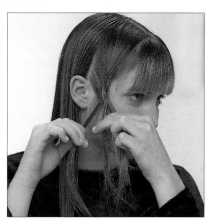

4 Continue down to the ends of the hair and secure with a small covered band. Repeat on the other side.

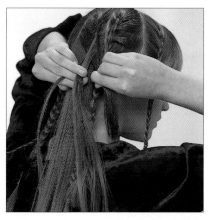

5 Part the back hair into four equal sections, from the crown down to the nape, and braid as shown. Start the braid at the top with three strands of hair and, after each turn of the braid, add a small section from each side.

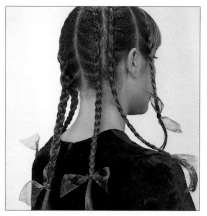

6 Secure the ends of the braids with small covered bands and decorate the braids with ribbon bows.

Band Braid

Aplain ponytail can be transformed beyond recognition by simply covering the band with a tiny braid.

Styling Checklist
Time: 5 minutes
Ease/difficulty: Easy
Hair type: Long, one length
You will need:
styling brush
styling wax
small covered band
hair grips

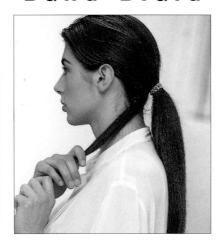

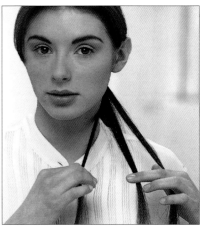

1 Brush the hair into a ponytail and secure with a band, leaving a small section free for braiding. Smooth the section with styling wax.

2 Divide this section into three equal strands. Now, braid the hair in the normal way.

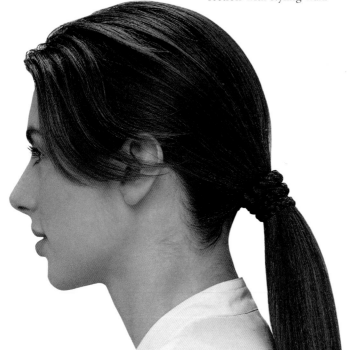

3 Take the braid and wrap it around the covered band as many times as it goes. Secure the braid in place with hair grips.

Draped Chignon

This elegant style is perfect for that special evening out.

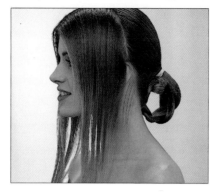

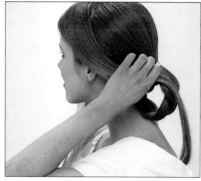

2 Loosely braid the ponytail – take the right strand over the centre strand, the left over the right, the right over the centre, and so on, continuing to the end. Secure the end with a small band, then tuck the end under and around in a loop and secure with grips.

3 Pick up the hair on the left side and comb it in a curve back to the ponytail loop. Swirl this hair over and under the loop and secure with grips. Repeat step 3 on the right side.

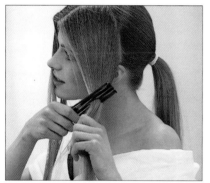

1 Part the hair in the centre from the forehead to the middle of the crown. Comb the side hair and scoop the back hair into a low ponytail using a covered band.

Tip
Long hair should be trimmed at least every two months to keep it in good condition.

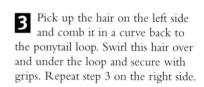

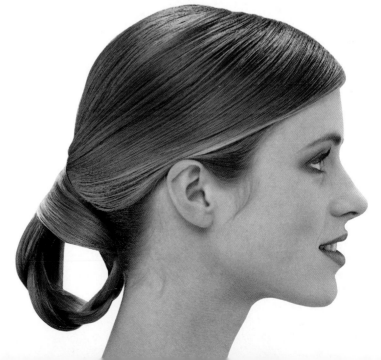

Simple Pleat

Curly hair that is neatly pleated makes a sophisticated style. The front is left full to soften the effect.

Styling Checklist
Time: 5 minutes
Ease/difficulty: Quite easy
Hair type: Shoulder length or longer
You will need:
serum
hairpins

1 Divide off a section of hair at the front and leave it free. Smooth with serum. Take the remaining hair into one hand, as if making a ponytail. Twist the hair tightly, the length of the ponytail, from left to right.

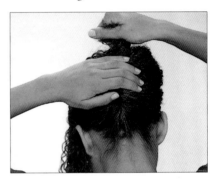

2 When the twist is taut, turn the hair upwards as shown to form a pleat. Use your other hand to help smooth the pleat and at the same time neaten the top by tucking in the ends.

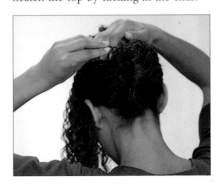

3 Secure the pleat with hairpins. Take the reserved front section, bring it back and secure at the top of the pleat, allowing the ends to fall free.

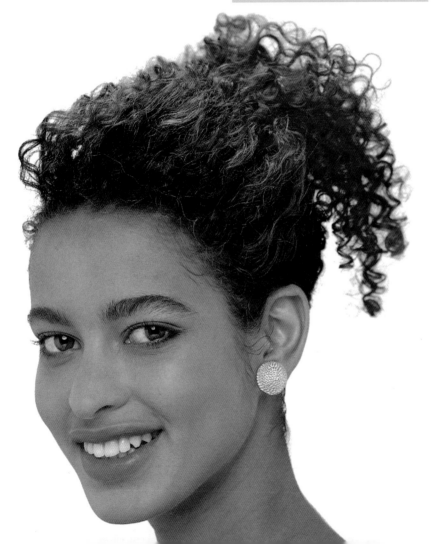

Looped Curls

Two ponytails form the basis of this elegant style.

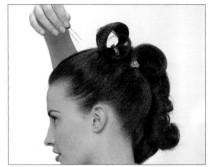

3 Divide each ponytail into sections about 2.5 cm/1 in wide, then comb and smooth each section into a looped curl and pin in place. Set with hairspray.

Tip
The speed at which rollers heat up depend on the type of roller, so check the instructions of your own model.

1 Apply setting lotion to the ends of the hair to help form bouncy curls. Set the hair on heated rollers for the required amount of time. When the rollers are cool – about 10 minutes after completing the set – take them out and allow the hair to fall free.

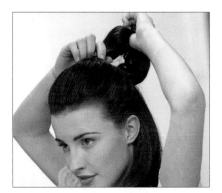

2 Divide off the crown hair and secure it with hair pins in a high ponytail. Apply a few drops of serum to add gloss, and brush the hair through. Place the remaining hair in a lower ponytail.

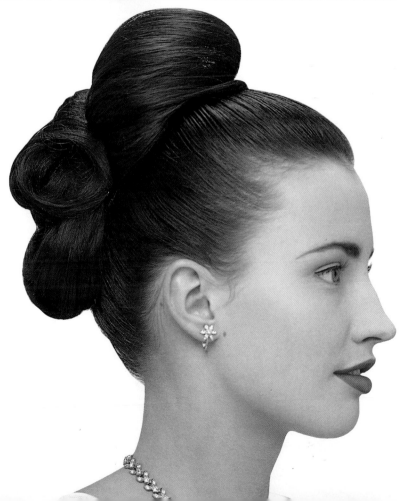

French Pleat

Mid-length to long hair can be transformed into a classic, elegant French pleat in a matter of minutes.

Styling Checklist
Time: 5–10 minutes
Ease/difficulty: Quite easy
Hair type: Mid-length to long
You will need:
styling comb
hair grips
hairpins
hairspray

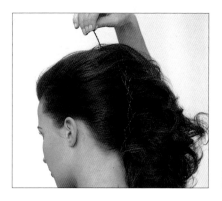

1 Backcomb the hair all over, then smooth it across to the centre back. Form the centre by criss-crossing hair grips from the crown downwards.

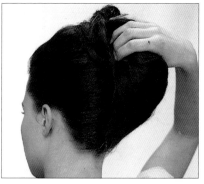

2 Gently smooth the hair around from the other side, leaving the front section free, and tuck the ends under to neaten.

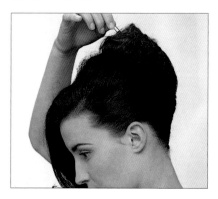

3 Secure with pins, then lightly comb the front section up and around to merge with the top of the pleat. Mist with hairspray to hold the style in place.

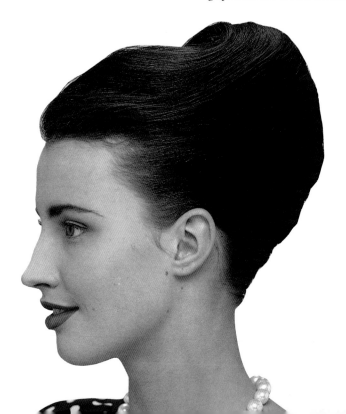

Short and Spiky

Short hair can be quickly styled using gel and wax to create a bold and fun look for instant glamour.

Styling Checklist

Time: 10 minutes
Ease/difficulty: Easy
Hair type: Short, layered and straight
You will need:
styling gel
hairdryer
styling comb
styling wax

1 Work styling gel through your hair from the roots to the ends.

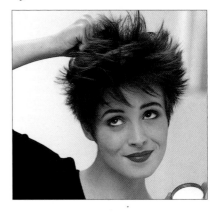

3 When the hair is dry, backcomb the crown to give additional height.

4 To finish, rub a little wax between the palms of your hands, then apply it to the hair to give definition.

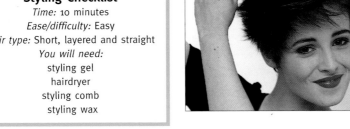

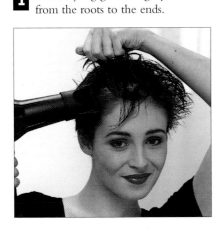

2 Dry your hair using a directional nozzle on your dryer; as you dry, lift sections of the hair to create height.

Tip

Gel can be reactivated by misting the hair with water and shaping it into style again.

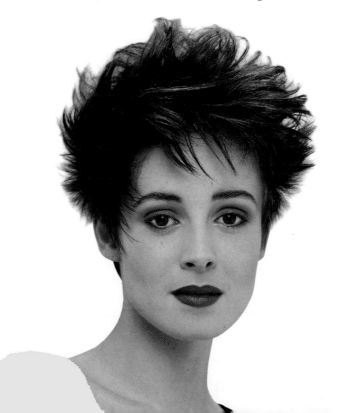

Accessories

Nothing becomes a hairstyle quite like hair accessories. Bandeaux, ribbons and bows come into their own at party time, but they can also be used at any time to transform your hair – instantly.

MAKE YOUR OWN

Some pretty fabrics and materials for hair accessories can be found in haberdashery departments of large stores. Look out for strips of sequins and pearls, or choose pretty ribbons, multi-coloured beads and tiny embroidered flowers that can be tied or simply pinned into place.

SCRUNCHIES

Scrunchies are elasticated bands that are covered with a tube of fabric, which ruches up when it is placed over a pony-tail. They are available in a wide variety of fabrics, including fine pleated silks, velvets and soft chiffons, so you can wear them to match your outfit.

BEADS

Beads can be threaded on to strands of hair and secured with small bands for special looks. You could revamp old clips and slides by adding your own beads to make some fun and original accessories.

BENDIES

Bendies are long pieces of flexible wire encased in fabric – often velvet or silk – that can be twisted into the hair in a variety of eye-catching ways; for example as a band, braided into a ponytail, entwined round a bun, or bound on to a braid. They come in many different colours and materials.

FLOWERS

For special occasions such as weddings, fresh flowers attached to clips make the perfect decoration. If you want to keep your floral accessories for longer, use silk flowers instead.

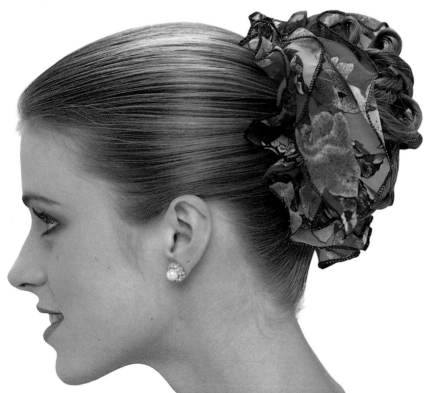

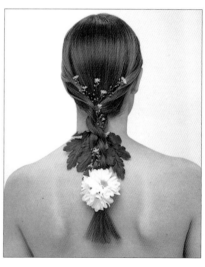

Above: Fresh flowers can be pinned into any braided style.

Left: A scrunchie completely alters the appearance of the Twist and Coil style.

BOWS

Bows can be tailored or floppy and are usually made from soft silks and velvets attached to a slide. Bows are available in a wide range of colours and designs.

HEADBANDS

Headbands come in a wide variety of fabrics and widths. Classic colours such as black, navy, red, cream and tortoise-shell are good basics.

SLIDES, CHIGNON PINS, COMBS

Unusual slides and barrettes are excellent for finishing off a braid or adding interest to a ponytail. Chignon pins add instant sophistication and are a means of securing buns. Combs can be used to lift the hair off the face, allowing the hair to fall free, but not in your eyes.

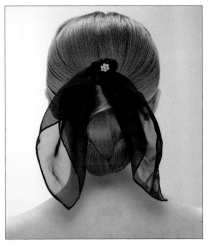

Above: A floppy bow adds instant sparkle to the Ponytail Styler.

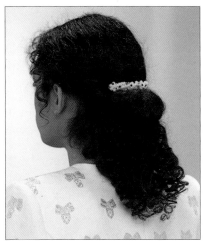

Above: A pearl slide gives added interest to the Curly Styler.

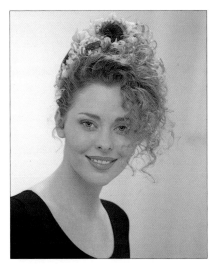

Above: Pin artificial flowers on top of an upswept style or into loosely styled curly hair for a young and very natural look.

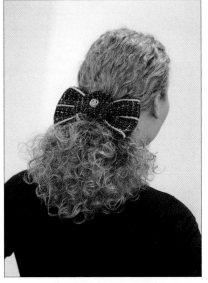

Above: For a very feminine touch add a pretty bow slide.

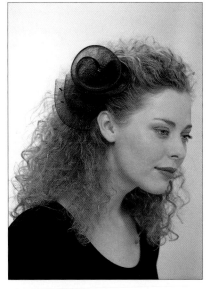

Above: For the evening, clip a classic bow among the curls.

Make-up Magic

The key to making-up successfully is to understand how to enhance your features, using the best cosmetic formulations and colours around. This doesn't mean spending a small fortune on the latest season's colours and promotions. Instead, it means analyzing what will work for you, your colouring and your lifestyle, then making your purchases. If you wise up on the best of the products, brush up your application techniques and give yourself time to experiment, you can find the perfect look for you. And, once you've mastered the basics, you can solve your own particular beauty problems, and try out some inspirational make-up ideas – just for fun!

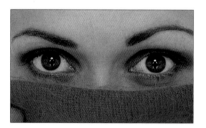

Above: Every woman can use make-up to emphasize her best features.

Right: Experiment with different styles to find the look that's right for you.

A Fabulous Foundation

Many women avoid wearing foundation because they're scared of an unnatural, mask-like effect. In fact, finding the right product for you is simpler than you might think. There are two keys to success: the first is to choose the perfect shade and the second is to pick the right formulation for your skin. With this shade and formulation selection, you can get the best coverage for your particular skin-type.

Tinted moisturizers

These are a cross between a moisturizer and a foundation, as they'll soothe your skin while giving a little coverage. They're ideal for young or clear skins. They're also great in the summer, when you want a sheer effect or to even out a fading tan. Unlike other foundations, you can blend tinted moisturizers on with your fingertips.

Liquid foundations

These suit all but the driest skins. If you have oily skin or suffer from breakouts, look for an oil-free liquid foundation to cover affected areas without aggravating them.

Cream foundations

These are thick, rich and moisturizing, making them ideal for dry or mature skins. They have a fairly heavy texture, so blend them well into your skin with a damp cosmetic sponge.

Mousse foundations

Again these are quite moisturizing, and ideal for drier skins. To apply, dab a little onto the back of your hand, then dot onto your skin with a sponge.

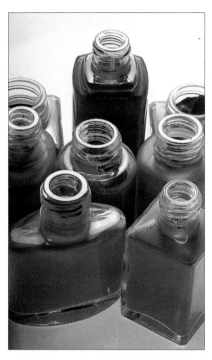

Above: Choose from a range of shades.

Compact foundations

These are all-in-one formulations, which already contain powder. They come in a compact, usually with their own sponge for application. They actually give a lighter finish than you'd expect.

Stick foundations

These are the original foundation, dating back to the early days of Hollywood. They have a heavy texture and so are best confined for use on badly blemished or scarred skin. Dot a little foundation directly onto the affected area, then blend gently with a damp sponge.

SHADE SELECTION

Once you've chosen the ideal formulation for you, you're ready to choose the perfect shade to match your skin.

■ Ensure you're in natural daylight when trying out foundation colours, so you can see exactly how your skin will look once you leave the shop or counter.

■ Select a couple of shades to try, which look as though they'll match your skin.

■ Don't try foundation on your hand or on your wrist – they're a different colour than your face.

■ Stroke a little colour onto your jawline to ensure you get a tone that will blend with your neck as well as your face. The shade that seems to "disappear" into your skin is the right one for you.

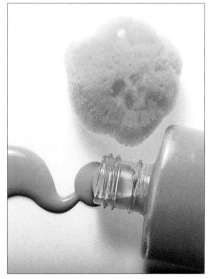

Above: Liquid foundation.

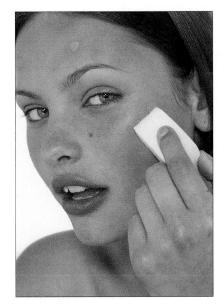

Above: Blend, blend, blend for a professional finish. And don't forget to give your face a final check to make sure you haven't got any unnatural lines where your foundation finishes.

APPLICATION KNOW-HOW

■ Apply foundation to freshly-moisturized skin to ensure you have a perfect base on which to work.

■ Use a cosmetic sponge to apply most types of foundation – using your fingertips can result in an uneven, greasy finish.

■ Apply foundation in dots, then blend each one with your sponge.

■ Dampen the sponge first of all, then squeeze out the excess moisture – this will prevent the sponge from soaking up too much costly foundation.

■ Check for "tidemarks" (streaks) on your jawline, nose, forehead and chin.

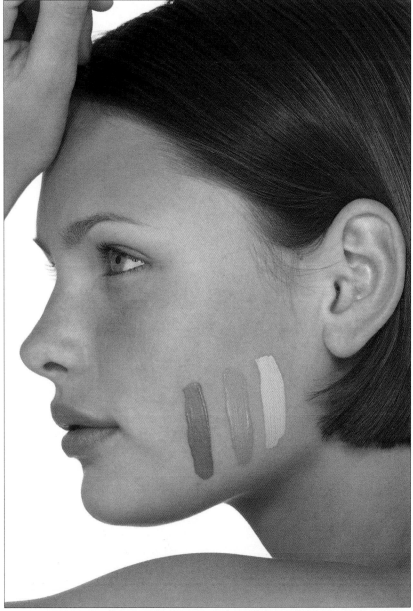

Above: Check different foundation colours on your jawline for the perfect match.

The Cover Up

Concealers are a fast and effective way to disguise blemishes, so your skin looks perfect. They're a concentrated form of foundation with a very high pigment content, so they offer complete coverage to problem areas. Applying them after foundation is best, as they are only applied to specific areas, and these would be disturbed if foundation is applied over the top.

Stick concealers

These are easy to apply as you can simply stroke them straight onto the skin. They're the most readily available type on the market. Some have quite a heavy and thick consistency, so it's worth trying out the different samples in the shop before you buy.

Cream concealers

These usually come in a tube, with a sponge-tipped applicator. The coverage isn't as thick as the stick type, but the finished effect is very natural.

Liquid concealers

Again, these come in a tube. Just squeeze a tiny amount of product onto your finger and smooth over the affected area. Look for the cream-to-powder formulations, which slick on like a cream and dry to a velvety powder finish.

Concealer Tip

When choosing a concealer look for the colour nearest to your own skin-tone rather than a lighter one. Covering a problem area with a paler shade will simply accentuate it.

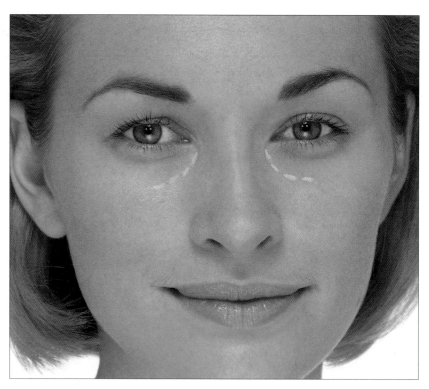

TAKING COVER

Here's how to conceal all your beauty problems effectively.

Spots and blemishes

The ideal solution is to use a medicated stick concealer as these contain ingredients to deal with the pimple or blemish as well as cover it. Only apply the concealer exactly on the pimple or blemish, as they can be quite drying, and then smooth away the edges with a clean cotton bud (swab). Applying concealer all around the area will make the spot more noticeable and create a "halo" effect.

Above: Hide under-eye shadows with a few dots of concealer. If you're after a light make-up effect, apply concealer directly onto clean skin, then apply powder or all-in-one foundation/powder over the top.

Under-eye shadows

Opt for a creamy stick concealer or a liquid one, as dry formulations will emphasize fine lines around your eyes. If you're blending with your fingertips, use your ring finger, as this is the weakest finger on your hand and less likely to drag at the delicate skin.

Pow! Wow! Powder!

Face powder is the make-up artist's best friend, as it can make your skin look really wonderful and is very versatile in its uses. Choose one that closely matches your skin-tone for a natural effect. Do this by dusting a little on your jawline, in the same way as you would with foundation.

■ Powder gives a super-smooth sheen to your skin – with or without foundation.

■ It "sets" your foundation, so it stays put and looks good for longer.

■ Powder absorbs oils from your skin, and helps prevent shiny patches.

■ It helps conceal open pores.

Loose powder

This gives the best and longest-lasting finish and is the choice of professional make-up artists and models. The best way to apply loose powder is to dust it lightly onto your skin using a large, soft powder brush. Then brush over your face again lightly to dust off the excess.

Pressed powder

Most come with their own application sponges, but you'll find you get a better result if you apply them with a brush. Look for brushes with retractable heads.

If you do use the sponge, use a light touch, and wash it regularly, or you'll transfer the oils in your skin onto the powder and get a build-up.

Above Right: Powder gives a perfect featherlight finish to your skin.

Right: Choose the shade that best suits your skin colouring.

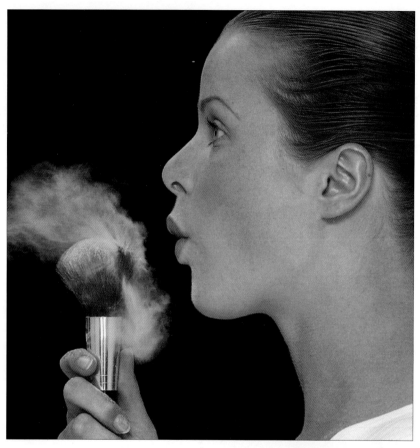

Powder Tip

When dusting excess powder away from your skin, use your brush in light, downward strokes to help prevent the powder from getting caught in the fine hairs on your skin. Pay particular attention to the sides of the face and jawline which aren't so easy for you to see.

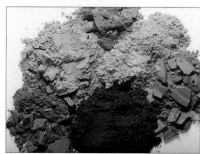

Blush Baby

Give your complexion a bloom of colour with this indispensable beauty aid.

Powder blusher

This should be applied over the top of your foundation and face powder. To apply powder blusher, dust over the compact with a large soft brush. If you've taken too much onto your brush, tap the handle on the back of your hand to remove the excess. It's better to waste a little blusher than apply too much!

Start the colour on the fullest parts of your cheeks, directly below the centre of your eyes. Then smile and dust the blusher over your cheekbones, and up towards your temples. Blend the colour well towards the hairline, so you avoid harsh edges. This will place colour where you would naturally blush.

Right: Brush your cheeks with colour.

Below: Be a blushing beauty with a light touch of powder blusher.

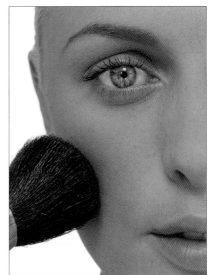

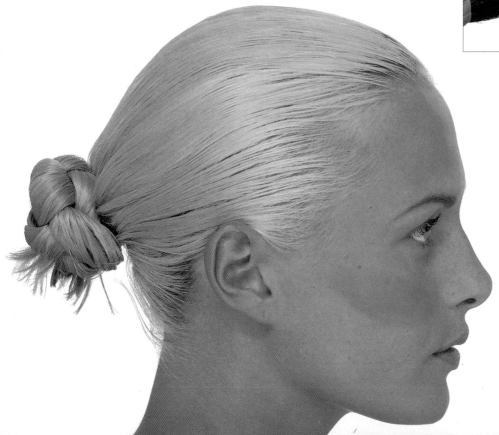

Cream blusher

Cream blusher is applied with your fingertips, after foundation, but before face powder. To apply, dab a few dots over your cheeks, from the plump part up towards your cheekbone. Using your fingertips, blend well. Build up the effect gradually, adding more blusher to create just the look you want. Or, if you prefer, you can use a foundation wedge to blend in cream blusher.

Colour choice

There's always a kaleidoscope of blusher shades to choose from. However, as a general rule, it's best to opt for a shade that tones well with your skin colouring, and co-ordinates with the rest of your make-up. You can opt for lighter or darker shades, depending on the season.

COLOUR GUIDE

Colouring	Choose
Blonde hair, cool skin	Pale pink shades
Blonde hair, warm skin	Pinky-brown shades
Dark hair, cool skin	Rose-pink shades
Dark hair, warm skin	Rose-brown shades
Red hair, cool skin	Pale peach shades
Red hair, warm skin	Warm peach shades
Dark hair, olive skin	Warm brown shades
Black hair, dark skin	Brown-red shades

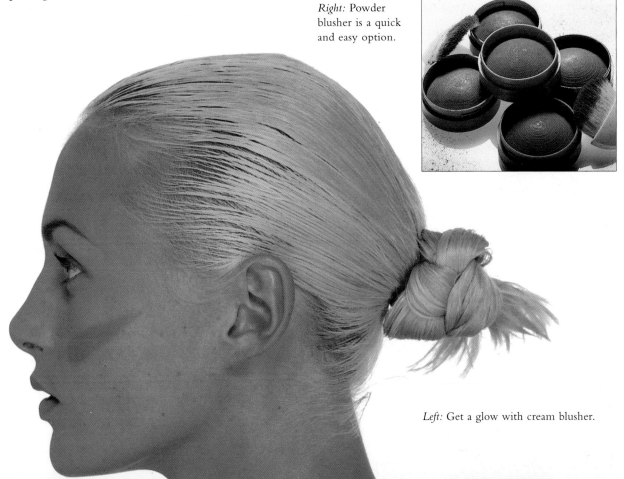

Right: Powder blusher is a quick and easy option.

Left: Get a glow with cream blusher.

The Eyes Have It

Eye make-up is the most popular type of cosmetic, and for good reason. Just the simplest touch of mascara can open up your eyes, while a splash of colour can transform them instantly. Whatever your eye shape and colour, you can ensure that they always look beautiful.

EYEBROW KNOW-HOW

Many women overlook their eyebrows, or sometimes even worse, overpluck them. When it comes to eye make-up, the eyebrows make an important impression. They can provide a balanced look to your face so it's well worth making the effort to get them looking right.

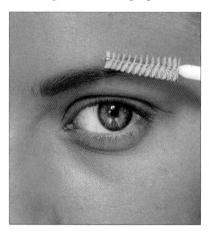

Natural brows
For perfectly groomed brows in an instant, try combing through them with a brush to flick away any powder or foundation. Comb the hairs upwards and outwards. This will also help give you a wide-eyed look. Then lightly slick them with clear gel to hold the shape neatly in place.

Eyebrow colour
To define your brows you can use eyebrow powder or pencil.

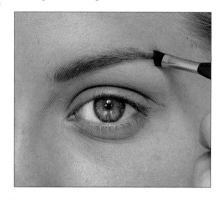

1 Apply powder with an eyebrow brush, dusting it through your brows and taking care not to sweep it onto the surrounding skin. This gives a natural effect, and requires little blending.

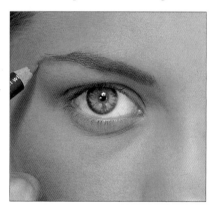

2 Alternatively, use a well-sharpened pencil to draw on tiny strokes, taking care not to press too hard or the finished effect will be unnatural.

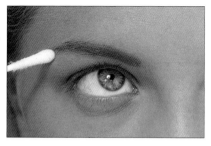

3 Then soften the lines you've made with the eye pencil by lightly stroking a clean cotton bud (swab) through your brows.

LINING UP LINER

Eyeliner is a great way to flatter all eye shapes and sizes. Eyeliner should be applied after eyeshadow and before your mascara.

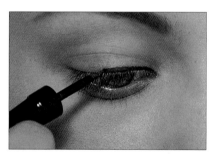

Liquid liners
These have a fluid consistency, and usually come with a brush attached to the cap. However, these aren't as easy to apply as the "ink-well" sponge-tipped variety. To apply the liner, look down into your mirror to prevent the liquid smudging. You should stay like this for a few seconds after applying the liner to give it time to dry thoroughly.

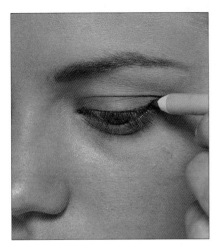

Pencil liners

This is the easiest way to add extra emphasis to your eyes. A pencil should be used to draw a line close to your upper and lower lashes. It's a good idea to sharpen the pencil between uses, not only to ensure you have a fine tip with which to work, but also to keep it bacteria-free.

Draw a soft line close to your lashes. If you find this quite difficult, try dotting it on along your lashes, then joining up the dots afterwards! Run over the pencil line with a brush. Alternatively, look for pencils that come with a smudger built in at the other end.

Eyeliner Know-How

If you've never applied liner before and feel a bit nervous, try this technique. Sit down at a table in a good light with a mirror. Take your eyeliner in your hand and rest your elbow on the table to keep your arm and hand steady. You can also give yourself extra support by resting your little finger on your cheek.

Eyeshadow as eyeliner

Make-up artists often use eyeshadow to outline the eyes, and it's a trick worth stealing! It looks great because it gives a very soft smoky effect.

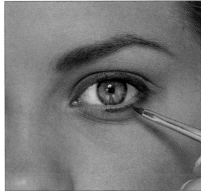

1 Use a small brush to apply shadow under your lower lashes and to make an impact over the top of the eyelid, taking care to keep the shadow close to the eyelashes.

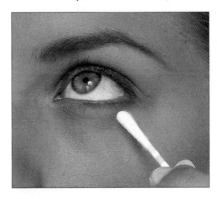

2 To create a softer, more modern effect simply sweep over the eyeshadow liner with a clean cotton bud (swab).

MASCARA MAGIC

Mascara adds a flattering fringe to your eyes – particularly if your lashes are fair.

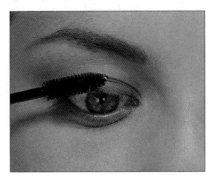

1 Start by applying mascara to your upper lashes first. Brush them downwards to start with, then brush your lashes upwards from underneath. Use a tiny zig-zag movement to prevent mascara from clogging on your lashes.

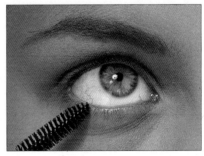

2 Next, use the tip of the mascara wand to brush your lower lashes, using a gentle side-to-side technique. Take care to keep your hand steady whilst you are applying the mascara, and not to blink whilst the mascara is still wet. Comb through your lashes with an eyelash comb to remove any excess the wand has left behind.

Below: Beautiful eyes – naturally.

Bottom Right: Experiment with different coloured powder shadows.

EYEING UP EYESHADOWS

Choose neutral colours to subtly enhance your looks, or play with a kaleidoscope of different shades to contrast with and dramatize your colouring.

Powder eyeshadows

The most popular type, these come in pressed cakes of powder either with a small brush or a sponge applicator. You can build up their density from barely-there to dramatic. Apply using a damp brush or sponge if you want a deep colour for an evening look.

Cream shadows

These are oil-based and come in little pots or compacts. They're applied either with a brush or your fingertips. They're a good choice for dry skins that need extra moisturizing.

Stick shadows

Wax-based, you smooth these onto your eyelids from the stick. Ensure they have a creamy texture before you buy them, so they won't drag at your skin.

Liquid shadows

Usually these come in a slim bottle with a sponge applicator. Look for the cream-to-powder ones that smooth on as a liquid and blend to a velvety powder finish.

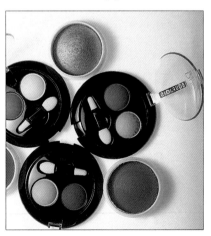

Brush Up Your Make-up

Even the most expensive make-up in the world won't look particularly great if it's applied carelessly and using your fingertips. For a professional finish you need the right tools. Here's your basic kit.

Make-up sponge

It is best to have a wedge-shaped make-up sponge, so you can use the finer edges to help blend in foundation round your nose and jawline, while the flatter edges are great for the cheeks, forehead and chin. However, if you prefer not to use a synthetic sponge you can try the small, natural ones instead.

Powder brush

Get used to using a powder brush each time you put make-up on. To prevent a caked or clogged finish to your face powder, use a large, soft brush to dust away any excess.

Blusher brush

Use to add a pretty glow to your skin with a light dusting of powder blusher. A blusher brush is slightly smaller than a powder brush to make it easier to control.

Eyeshadow brush

Smooth on any shade of eyeshadow with this brush.

Eyebrow tweezers

It is essential to have a good pair of tweezers for regularly tidying up the eyebrows.

Eyeshadow sponge

A sponge applicator is great for applying a sweep of pale eyeshadow that does not need much blending, or for applying highlighter to your brow bones.

All-in-one eyelash brush/comb

Great for combing through your lashes between coats of mascara for a clump-free finish. Flip the comb over and use the brush side to sweep your eyebrows into shape, or soften pencilled-in brows.

Lipbrush

Use to create a perfect outline for your lips and then use to fill in the shape with your lipstick.

Eyelash curlers

Once used, they'll soon become a beauty essential! Curlier eyelashes help open up your eyes and make a huge difference to the way you look.

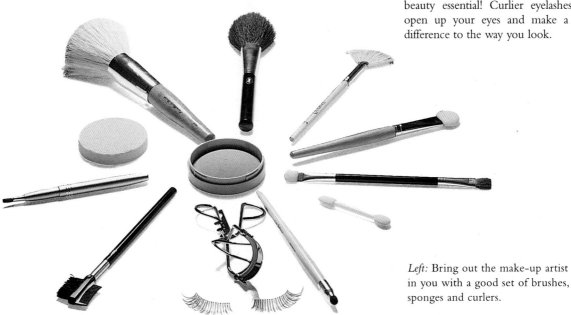

Left: Bring out the make-up artist in you with a good set of brushes, sponges and curlers.

Eye Make-up Masterclass

Now that you know where to start, you can experiment with more sophisticated eye make-up methods to create a variety of stunning looks. Here's a look you can try, using a wide range of techniques to create the ultimate in glamorous eye make-up.

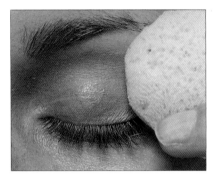

1 Smooth over your eyelids with foundation to create an even base on which to work, and to give your eye make-up something to cling to.

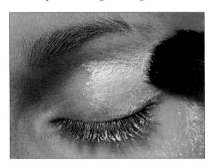

2 Sweep over your eyelids with a brush loaded with translucent face powder. Dust a little translucent powder under your eyes to catch any flecks of fallen eyeshadow later.

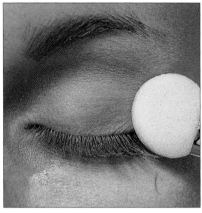

3 Use a sponge applicator to sweep a neutral ivory shade over your eyelids. Work it right up towards your eyebrows for a balanced overall effect.

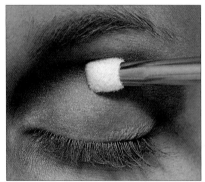

4 Smudge a brown eyeshadow into the socket line of your eyes, using a sponge applicator. If you find blending difficult, try using a slightly shimmery powder as these are easier to work in. Use a brush to sweep over the top of the brown shadow as this will remove any harsh edges.

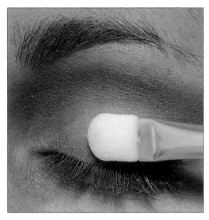

5 To create a perfectly blended finish, sweep some more ivory shadow over the edges of the brown eyeshadow using a sponge applicator. Now that you've completed your eyeshadow, flick away the powder from under your eyes.

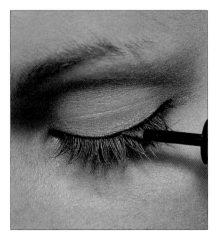

6 Looking down into a mirror and keeping your hand steady, apply liquid eyeliner along your upper lashes.

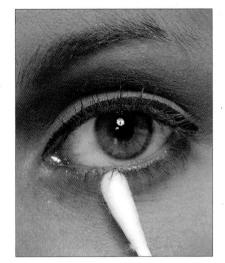

7 Use a clean cotton bud (swab) to work some brown eyeshadow under your lower lashes to add some subtle definition.

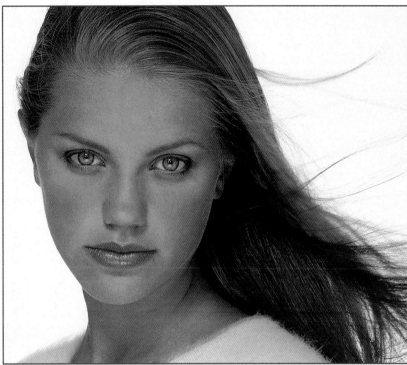

Above: For our main look here, we used a palette of ivory and blue eyeshadow, combined with black eyeliner and mascara. Take time to experiment with different colours to find a look that suits you and your colouring.

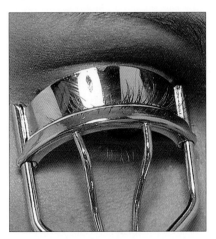

8 Squeeze your lashes with eyelash curlers to make them bend, before applying mascara. This will "open up" the eye area.

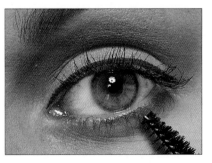

9 Apply mascara onto your upper lashes and use the tip of the mascara wand to coat your lower lashes.

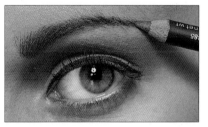

10 Stroke your eyebrows with pencil to shape them and fill in any patches. Smooth over the top with a cotton bud (swab) to soften the eyebrow pencil line.

Getting Lippy

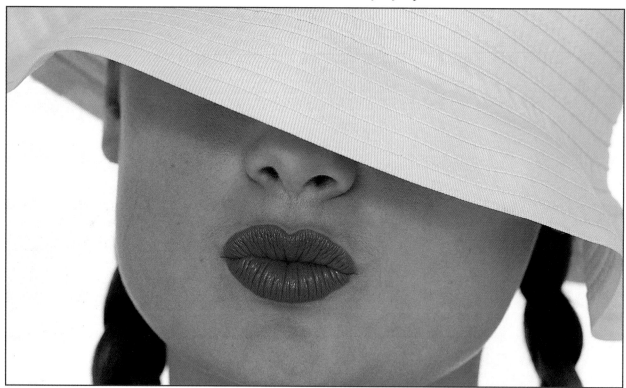

Lipstick has been around for about 5,000 years! It's the easiest and quickest way to give your face a focus and create an instant splash of colour.

A LICK OF COLOUR

■ Lipsticks in a bullet form are the most popular way to use lip colour. Some lipsticks even come with in-built Sun Protection sunscreens.

■ Another way of applying colour is with a lip gloss. These can be used alone to give your lips an attractive sheen, or over the top of lipstick to catch the light.

■ Lipliners are used to provide an outline to your lips before applying lipstick. You can also use them over your entire lip for a dark, matte effect. However, you may need to add a touch of lipsalve (balm) over the top to prevent drying out this delicate area of skin.

Above: A slick of colour will make you love your lips. The best way to apply lipstick is with a lipbrush.

Right: A selection of lipstick colours is the key to creating different looks.

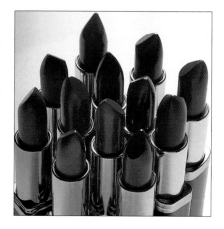

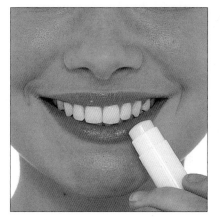

1 Ensure your lips are soft and supple by smoothing over moisturizer before you start.

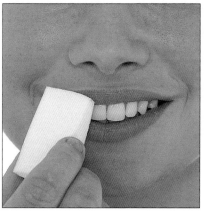

2 Prime your lips by smoothing them with foundation, using a make-up sponge so you reach every tiny crevice on the surface.

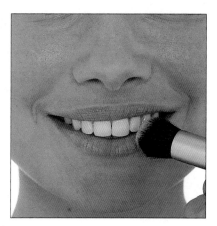

3 Dust over the top of the foundation with a light dusting of your usual face powder, to help your lipstick stay put for longer.

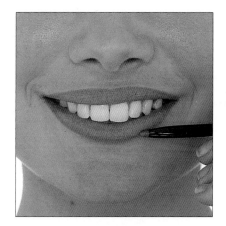

4 Rest your elbow on a firm surface and carefully draw an outline using a lip pencil. So it doesn't drag your skin, it may help to warm it slightly in your palm. Start by defining the Cupid's bow on the upper lip, then draw a neat outline on your lower lip. Finish by completing the edges of the outline to your upper lip.

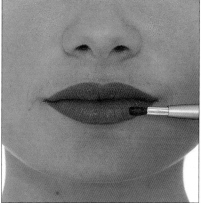

5 Use a lipbrush to fill in the outline with lipstick, ensuring you reach into every tiny crevice on the surface. Open your mouth to brush the colour into the corners of your lips.

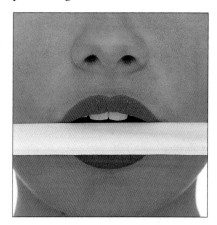

6 You'll help your lipstick last longer if you blot over the surface with a tissue. It'll also give an attractive, semi-matte finish to your lips. Reapply to help a longer-lasting finish.

Cool Skin, Blonde Hair

With your porcelain complexion and pale hair, you should opt for baby pastel tones with sheer formulations and a hint of shimmer. This way you'll flatter your colouring with a light, fresh make-up look, without overpowering it.

THIS LOOK SUITS YOU IF…

■ You have pale blonde to mousy or mid-blonde hair.

■ Your eyes are blue, grey, hazel or green.

■ You have pale skin, including whiter-than-white, ivory or a pinky "English rose" complexion.

Tip
If you're older, or unsure about wearing blue eyeshadow, swap it for a cool grey. This will create the same soft effect, but it's more subtle. You may prefer to switch to matte ivory instead of shimmery eyeshadow.

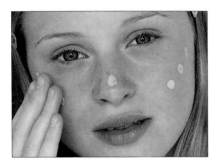

1 Your delicate skin doesn't need heavy coverage, so use a light tinted moisturizer. Dot it lightly onto your nose, cheeks, forehead and chin, then blend it in with your fingertips.

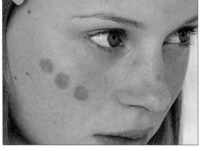

2 Cool pink blusher will give a soft glow to your skin. Dot onto your cheeks, then blend in with your fingertips. Either skip powder to leave your skin with a dewy glow, or gently dust a little over your face.

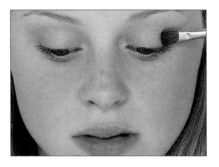

3 Take a baby blue eyeshadow onto an eyeshadow brush and sweep it evenly over your entire eyelid. Stroke the brush gently over your eyelid a few times until you've swept away any obvious edges to the eyeshadow.

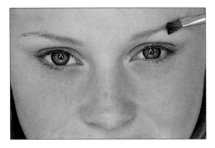

4 Sweep a shimmery ivory shadow from the crease in your eyelid up towards the brow bone to open up the eye area.

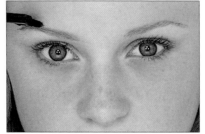

5 Stroke your eyebrow into shape with an eyebrow brush. This will also flick away any powder that's got caught in the hairs.

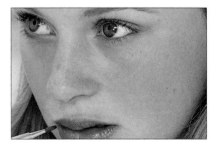

6 Cool pink lipstick should be applied with a lipbrush. If you like, you can slick a little lipgloss or lip balm on top for a sexy shimmer.

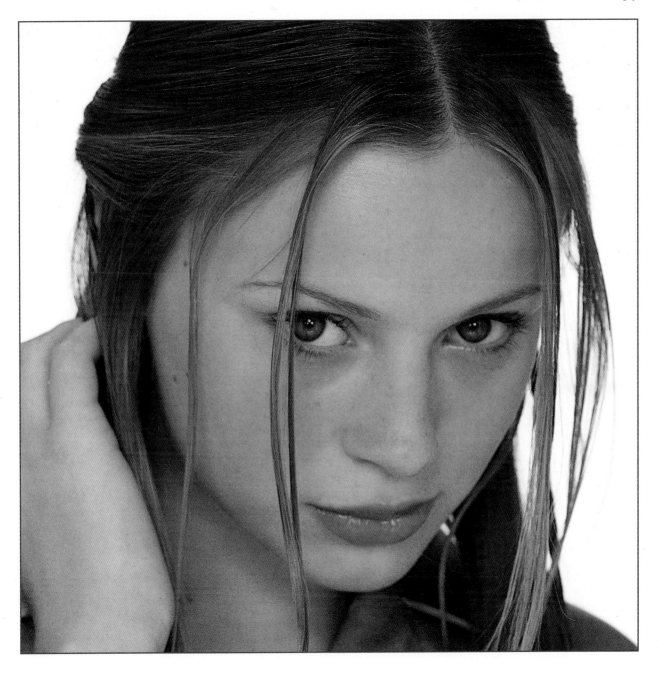

Warm Skin, Blonde Hair

Although you have a warm skin-tone, your overall look is quite delicate. This means you should opt for tawny, neutral shades of make-up, and apply them with a light touch so you enhance your basic colouring.

THIS LOOK SUITS YOU IF...

■ You have golden, warm blonde or dark blonde hair.

■ Your eyes are brown, blue, hazel or green – it will work equally well.

■ You have a warm skin-tone which can develop a light, golden tan.

■ Your skin tone and blonde hair mean your overall look is quite delicate. If so, you need to choose make-up shades that are not too intense, like those here.

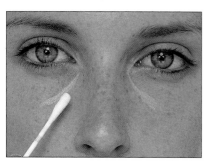

1 After applying a light, tinted moisturizer, stroke concealer onto problem areas. Blondes tend to have fine skin, often prone to surface thread veins. Cover these effectively with concealer, applied with a clean cotton bud (swab).

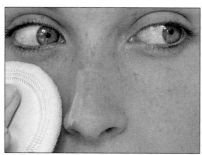

2 Dip a powder puff into loose powder and lightly press over the areas of your face that are prone to oiliness. This will absorb excess oil throughout the day, and leave your skin beautifully matte. Dust off any excess.

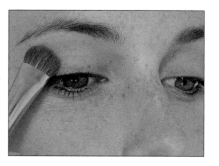

3 Sweep peach eyeshadow over your entire eyelid. It will blend with your natural skin-tone, but give a clean, wide-eyed look to your make-up.

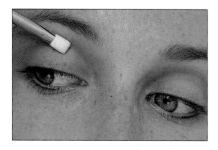

4 Use an eyeshadow brush to work a tiny amount of soft brown eyeshadow into the crease of your eyelid to create depth and definition to your eyes. Sweep it out towards the outer corner of your eyes as well.

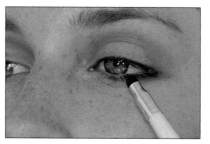

5 Still using the same brown eyeshadow, work a little underneath your lower lashes. This gives a softer effect than traditional kohl pencil or eyeliner. Finish with two coats of brown/black mascara.

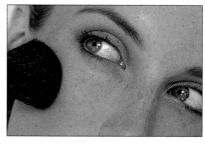

6 Apply a light shade of lipstick. Then apply your blusher, sweeping it a little at a time over your cheeks, forehead and chin. You can even dust a little over the tip of your nose!

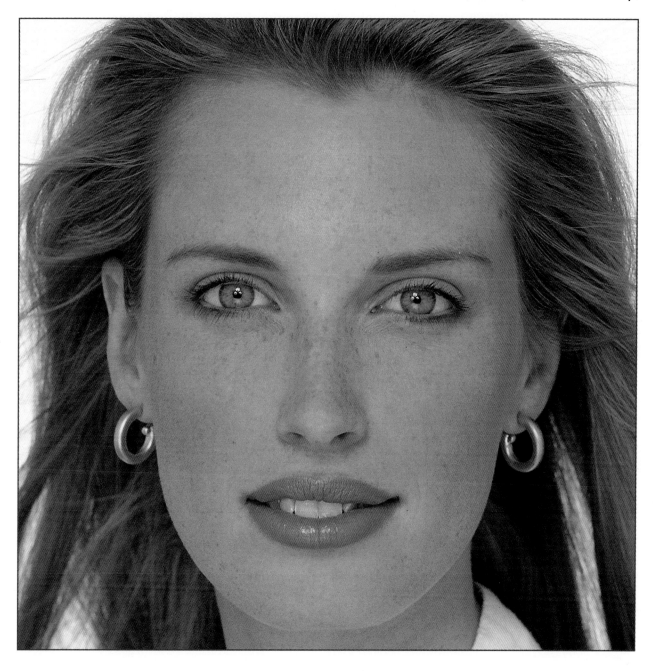

Cool Skin, Dark Hair

Pale-skinned brunettes look fabulous with strong, cool shades of cosmetics. The density of colour provides a striking contrast to ivory skin-tones, while their coolness tones in beautifully with your natural beauty.

THIS LOOK SUITS YOU IF....

■ You have medium to dark brown hair.

■ Your eyes are brown, blue, grey or green.

■ You have a cool, China doll skin-tone, that tans slowly in the sun.

Tip
To stop your mascara from clogging, wiggle the mascara wand from side to side as you pull it through your lashes.

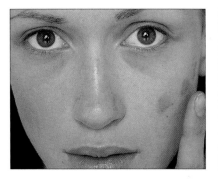

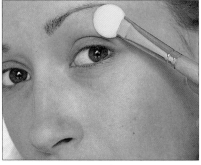

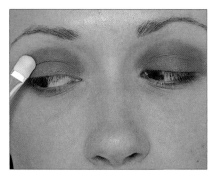

1 Apply foundation or tinted moisturizer. Whichever you use, it's likely you'll need the palest of shades. Blend in a few dots of blusher. Dust with loose powder.

2 Smudge a cool ivory shadow over your eyelids, right up to your eyebrows. Stroke over it with a cotton bud (swab) to blend it if you find it gathers in creases.

3 Add extra definition with a touch of mocha eyeshadow on your eyelids. This shade works beautifully on your cool colouring, and emphasizes the colour of your eyes.

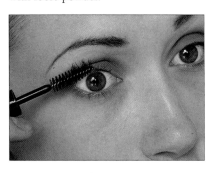

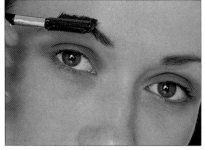

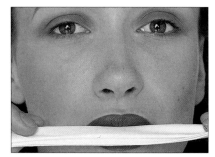

4 Now move onto your eyelashes. You need to apply two thin coats of black mascara to create a wonderful frame to your eyes.

5 Slick your eyebrows into place with an eyebrow brush. If they tend to look untidy, hold them in place by spritzing the brush with a little hairspray first.

6 Choose a clear shade of berry lipstick to give your look a polished finish. Blot after one coat with a tissue, then re-apply to help a longer-lasting finish.

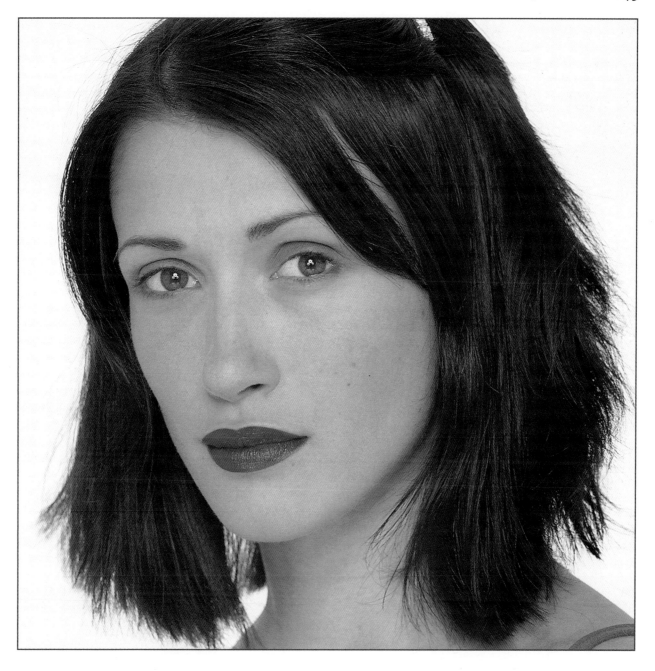

Warm Skin, Dark Hair

Your skin-tone can carry off burnished browns, warm reds and earthy shades beautifully. They'll complement your complexion and emphasize your features.

THIS LOOK SUITS YOU IF...

■ You have mid to dark brown hair.

■ Your eyes are brown, dark blue, grey, hazel or green.

■ You have a warm skin-tone that usually tans quite well. Even if it is pale in winter, your skin probably still has a yellow undertone.

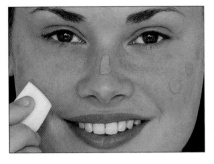

1 Dot liquid foundation onto your skin and blend in with a damp cosmetic sponge. Blend the colour into your neckline for a natural effect. Then apply concealer to any blemishes.

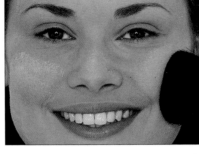

2 Pat your face with translucent loose powder, then fluff off the excess with a large, soft brush.

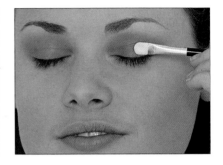

3 Use a sponge-tipped eyeshadow applicator to sweep a red-brown shadow over your entire eyelid. The advantage of the sponge over a brush is that it doesn't flick colour around.

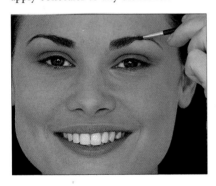

4 Your eyebrows need subtle emphasis for this look. Either pencil them in with soft strokes of brown eyebrow pencil, or use a brown eyeshadow for a softer effect. Brush and then slick the hairs in place.

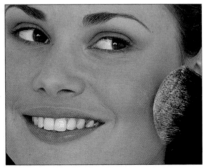

5 Opt for a warm, tawny brown shade of powder blusher, dusted over your cheeks and up towards your temples. As this colour is quite strong, you may need to tone it down a little with translucent loose powder.

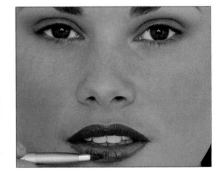

6 A fiery red lipstick balances the overall look. Use a lipbrush to ensure you fill in every tiny crease and crevice on the lip surface – this can help your lipstick colour stay put for longer as well as create a perfect finish.

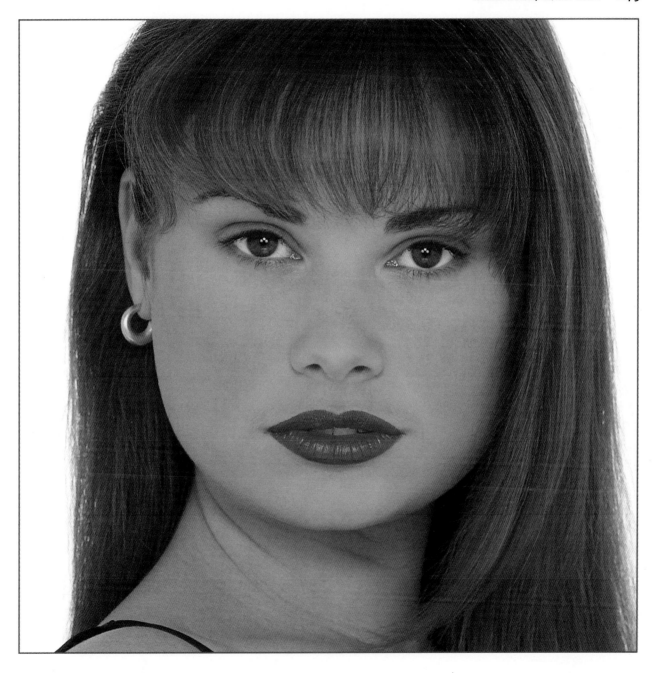

Cool Skin, Red Hair

Redheads with cool skin-tones often stick to wishy-washy colours, but you can experiment with brighter colours to contrast with your wonderful colouring. Greens give an exciting dimension to your eyes, and strong earthy shades supercharge your lips.

THIS LOOK SUITS YOU IF...

▪ You have strawberry-blonde or pale red hair, even if the colour has faded.

▪ Your eyes are blue, grey, hazel or green.

▪ You have pale skin, ranging from ivory to a pink-toned complexion.

Tip
If you've got freckles, don't fall into the trap of trying to cover them with a dark-toned foundation. Instead, match your foundation to your skin-tone to avoid a mask-like effect.

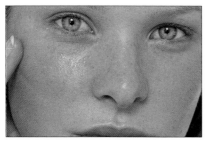

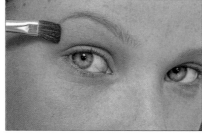

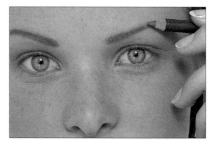

1 Apply foundation and concealer, then dot a peachy shade of blusher onto your cheekbones. Apply a little blusher at a time, and add more if you need it. Finish with loose powder.

2 A neutral, peach-toned eyeshadow swept over your eyelids will emphasize your eye colour without fighting with it. Ensure you take care to work it close to your eyelashes.

3 Opt for a very pale eyebrow pencil, in a subtle grey-brown tone. Stroke it through your eyebrows, taking care to fill any bald spots. Then soften the lines with an eyebrow brush.

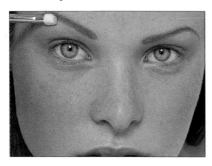

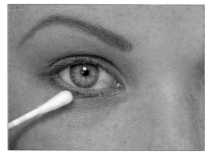

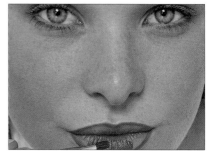

4 Brush a hint of gold, shimmery eyeshadow into the arch under your eyebrows to give your eyes an extra dimension. This is a good way to bring out gold flecks or warmth in the irises of your eyes.

5 Work green eyeliner along your upper lashes and into the corners of your eyes as well. Smudge over the top to give a softer finish. Brush over a little translucent powder and complete with two thin coats of brown mascara.

6 Burnished orange lipstick complements this look. Begin by outlining your lips with a toning lip liner to help prevent the colour from bleeding. Then use a lipbrush to fill in with the lipstick.

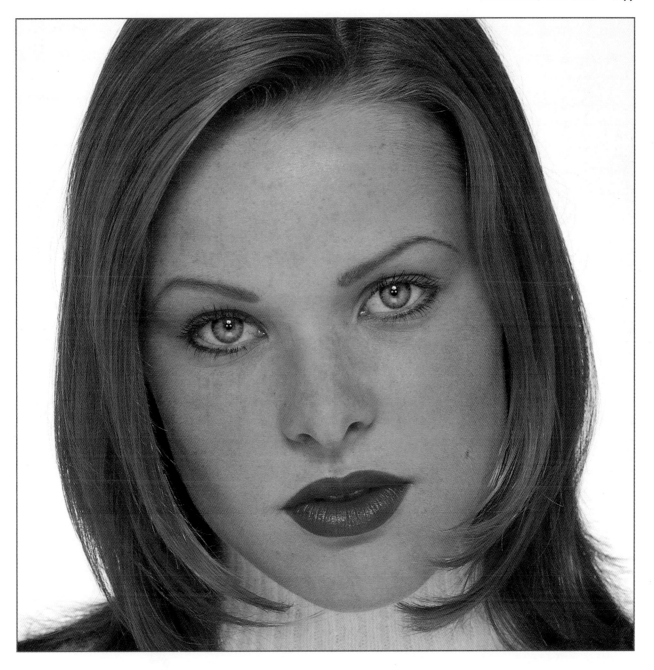

Warm Skin, Red Hair

Your vibrant Pre-Raphaelite colouring is suited to bold shades of wine, purple and brown. These deep, blue-toned colours look fabulous with your warm skin and hair tones, and can make you look truly stunning.

THIS LOOK SUITS YOU IF...

■ You have medium to dark red hair. This look may also suit brunettes who have a lot of red tones to their hair.

■ Your eyes are blue, grey, brown or green.

■ You have a medium to warm skin-tone.

■ Your skin takes on a golden colour in the summer, although you're unlikely to get a deep tan. It's quite likely that you have freckles.

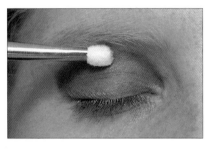

1 After applying foundation, concealer and powder, smooth a wine shade of shadow over your entire eyelid. Using a sponge-tipped eyeshadow applicator will give you more control.

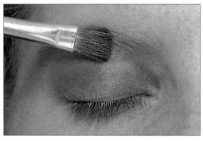

2 Use a pale mauve eyeshadow over your brow bone to balance your eye make-up. Blend it into the crease, to soften any harsh edges of the wine-toned eyeshadow. Take your time at this stage, for a professional-looking finish.

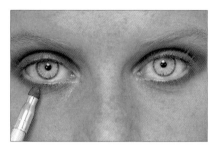

3 Smudge a little eyeshadow under your lower lashes as well. Work it into the outer corners, sweeping it slightly upwards to give your eyes a lift. Then finish with two coats of brown mascara.

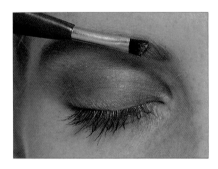

4 Use a soft brown eyeshadow on your eyebrows to give them subtle emphasis, using either a small brush, or a cotton bud (swab). Brush the eyebrows through afterwards with an eyebrow brush for a soft finish.

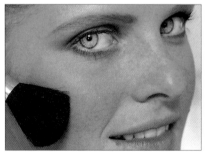

5 Choose a brown-toned blusher or bronzing powder to give your skin lots of warmth. Dust it on with a large blusher brush, blending it out towards your hairline for a natural glow. The key is to use a little at a time.

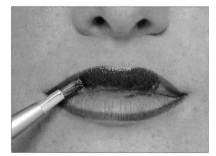

6 You can carry off a deep plum shade of lipstick, outlined with a toning lip pencil. This strong colour needs perfect application to look good, so apply two coats, blotting in between with a tissue.

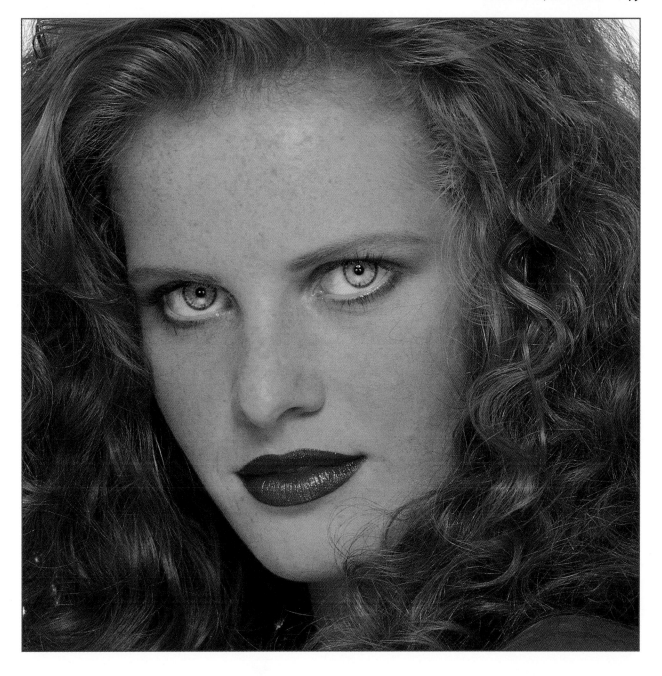

Olive Skin, Dark Hair

Your skin-tones are easy to complement with rich browns, oranges and a hint of gold or bronze. These rich shades define your features and work well on your wonderful skin-tones.

THIS LOOK SUITS YOU IF...

■ You have dark brown to black hair.

■ Your eyes are brown, hazel or green.

■ Your olive skin tans beautifully, or you have Asian or Indian colouring.

Tip

To create a perfect lip line, stretch your mouth into an "O" shape and fill in the corners with your lip pencil.

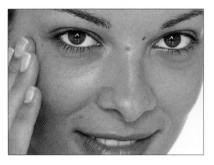

1 Even out minor skin blemishes with a tinted moisturizer, blending it in with fingertips. If you need more coverage, opt for a liquid or cream foundation. Now apply a concealer and a light dusting of face powder.

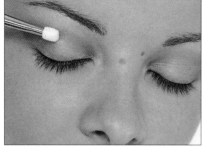

2 After sweeping a golden shade of shadow across your entire eyelid, apply a darker bronze shade into the crease and then apply some under the lower lashes. This gives a wonderfully sultry look to your eyes.

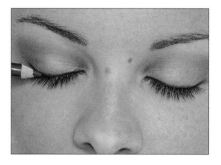

3 Take a warm brown eyeliner, and work it along your upper and lower lashes for a strong look that you can carry off beautifully. If you find the effect too harsh, lightly stroke over the top with a clean cotton bud (swab).

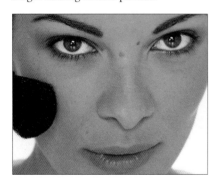

4 A peach-brown powder blusher adds a sunkissed warmth to your cheeks. Apply just a little at a time, increasing the effect as you go.

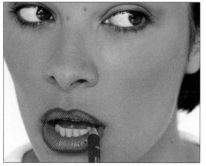

5 Outline your lips with an orange-brown lip pencil. Start at the Cupid's bow on the upper lip, and move out. Finish with the lower lip.

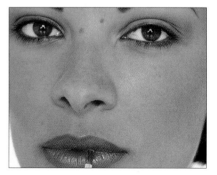

6 To complete the look, fill in with a sunny orange shade of lipstick. If you like a glamorous, glossy finish, don't blot your lips with a tissue.

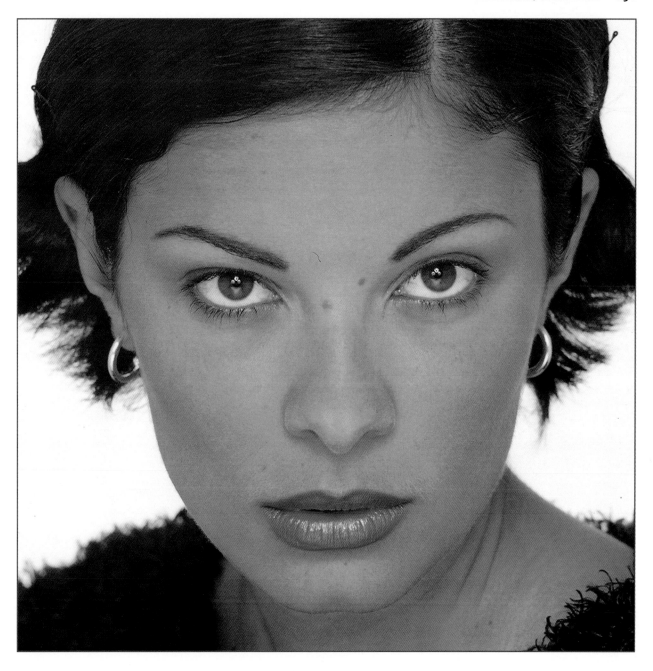

Olive Skin, Asian Colouring

Your black hair, and pale – but yellow-toned – skin are best complemented by soft, warm colours. These will define your looks and counteract any sallowness in your complexion.

THIS LOOK SUITS YOU IF...

- You have dark brown to black hair.
- Your eyes are hazel or brown.
- You have a pale to medium skin-tone.

Tip
Asian eyelashes are often poker-straight and so you can really benefit from the use of eyelash curlers.

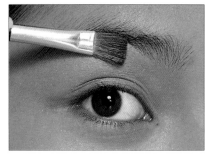

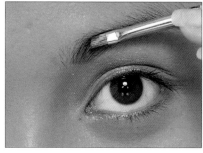

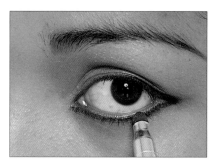

1 After applying your foundation, concealer and powder, sweep some lilac eyeshadow over your eyelid. This pale colour is a better option than using darker eyeshadows near the eyes as they have a tendency to make them look deep set, particularly as your eyelids tend to be quite small.

2 Lightly fill in your eyebrows with a dark brown eyeshadow or eyebrow pencil to provide a strong frame to your eyes. This will help balance the eyeliner which is going to be applied next.

3 A lick of blue-black eyeliner will emphasize your beautifully-shaped eyes, and help correct any droopiness. Slick it along the lower lashes and into the outer corners of your eyes to create balance. To prevent the overall look from seeming too harsh, use a cotton bud (swab) to soften the eyeliner slightly.

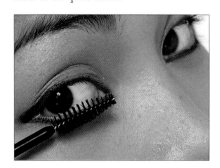

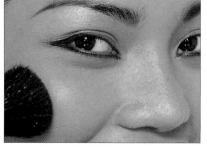

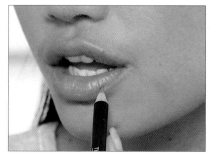

4 Place your eyelashes between the edges of a curler, and gently squeeze for a few seconds. Then apply two coats of black mascara.

5 A warm pink blusher gives a wonderful boost to your complexion and brings out its natural glow. Dust it over the plumpest part of your cheeks.

6 A baby pink lipliner and lipstick bring your lips fashionably into focus. The cool blue tone to this shade works wonderfully on your colouring.

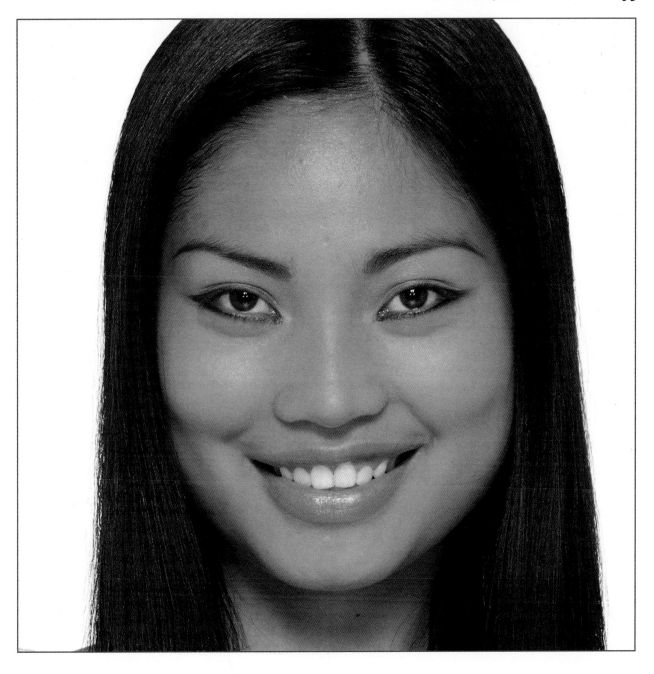

Black Hair, Pale Black Skin

Try emphasizing your looks with rich earthy shades. Your gold or red-toned skin works wonderfully with beige, brown and copper colours.

THIS LOOK SUITS YOU IF...

- ■ You have black hair with highlights.
- ■ Your have hazel or brown eyes.
- ■ You have black skin.

Tip

Look at cosmetic ranges especially designed for darker skins for your foundation and powder.

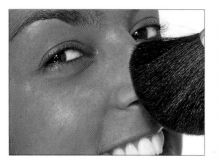

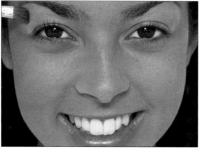

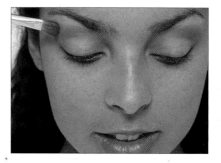

1 After applying foundation, dust on a translucent face powder, ensuring it perfectly matches your skin-tone to avoid a chalky looking complexion. Dust off the excess with a large powder brush, using downward strokes.

2 Use an eyeshadow brush to dust an ivory-toned eyeshadow over your entire eyelid, to create a contrast with your warm skin-tone.

3 Smudge a deep-toned brown eyeshadow into the crease of your eyelid, blending it thoroughly. Also work a little of this colour into the outer corners and underneath your lower lashes to make your eyes look really striking.

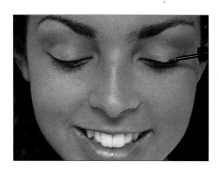

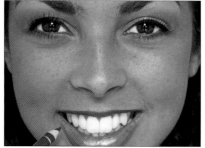

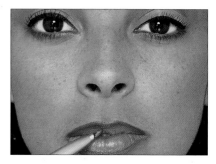

4 Sweep black liquid eyeliner along your upper lashes whilst looking down into a mirror, as this stretches creases out of your eyelid. Follow with two coats of black mascara.

5 Use a brown lipliner pencil to outline your lips. (Use a brown eyeliner pencil if you don't have a lipliner pencil.) Blend in the line, using a cotton bud (swab) for a softer effect.

6 A neutral pink-brown lipstick gives a natural looking sheen to your lips and instantly updates your looks. Apply lipstick with a lipbrush for a perfectly even finish.

Black Hair, Deep Black Skin

You can experiment with endless colour possibilities as your dark eyes, hair and skin provide the perfect canvas on which to work. The key to success is to choose bold, deep colours as these will give your skin a wonderful glow.

THIS LOOK SUITS YOU IF...

■ You have deep black hair, even if it has flecks of grey.

■ You have dark hazel or brown eyes.

■ You have a dark black skin.

> **Tip**
> While dramatic colours suit your skin-tone and colouring perfectly, be sure to apply them with a light touch to get a fresh, up-to-date look.

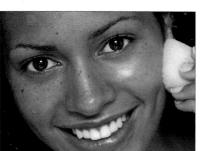

1 Choose a foundation that matches your skin-tone exactly. Apply the foundation with a damp sponge, blending it along your jaw and hairline to avoid "tidemarks" (streaks). Finally, set with a light dusting of translucent loose powder.

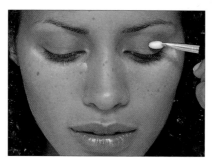

2 Next, sweep a dark blackcurrant eyeshadow over your eyelids. Dust a little loose powder under your eyes first to catch any falling specks of this dark shade, and prevent it from ruining your completed foundation.

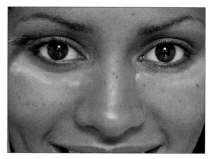

3 Apply a dark charcoal eyeshadow into the crease of your eyelid, using an eyeshadow brush. Take only a little colour at a time to the brush to prevent it from spilling on to your eyelid. If necessary, tap the brush on the back of your hand first to shake away any excess.

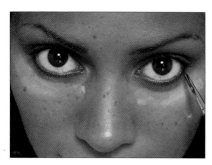

4 Use an eyeliner brush to work under your lower lashes. Hold the mirror above your eyeliner for accuracy. Finish with two coats of black mascara.

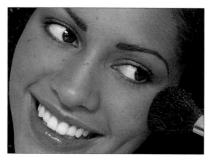

5 Choose a tawny brown shade of blusher to complement your skin. With a large brush, dust over your cheeks, working towards the hairline.

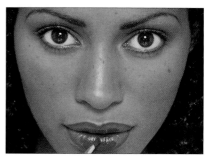

6 After outlining your lips with a toning lip pencil, fill in with a dark plum shade of lipstick, using a lipbrush.

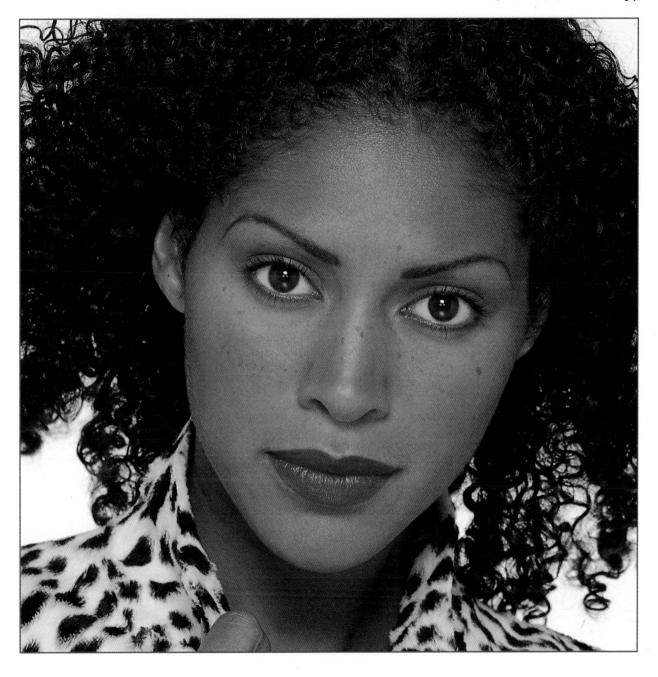

The Five-Minute Face

When you haven't got time to spare, try this quick routine for evening sophistication. The key is to choose simple looks, applied with a minimum of fuss when you're racing the clock... in other words, simple steps to a sexy look!

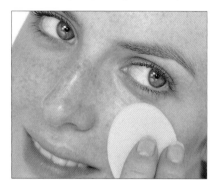

Five minutes to go...

The all-in-one foundation-powder formulations give your skin the medium coverage it needs for this look in half the time. Take it over lips and eyelids.

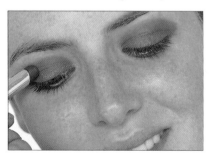

Four minutes to go...

Cream eyeshadow applied straight from the stick is quick and easy to apply. Opt for a brown shade as it'll bring out the colour of your eyes and give them a sexy, sultry finish. Slick it over your entire eyelid.

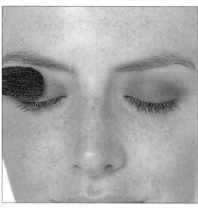

Three and a half minutes to go...

A swift way to blend in your eyeshadow is to brush over the top with translucent loose powder. This will tone down the colour and blend away any harsh edges.

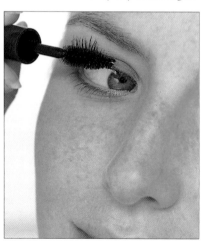

Two and a half minutes to go...

Apply a coat of mascara to your lashes, taking care to colour your lower lashes as well as your upper ones. Use the tip of the mascara wand to coat the lower lashes.

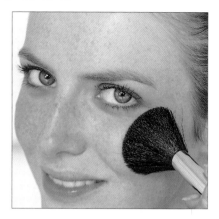

One and a half minutes to go...

A warm berry red blusher will give your skin a fabulous flush. Apply it with a blusher brush, sweeping it from your cheeks up towards your eyes.

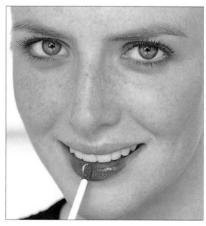

Thirty seconds to go...

Choose a berry shade of lipstick to add instant bold colour to your lips, sweeping it straight on. Cover your lower lip first, then press your lips together to transfer some of the colour onto your upper lip.

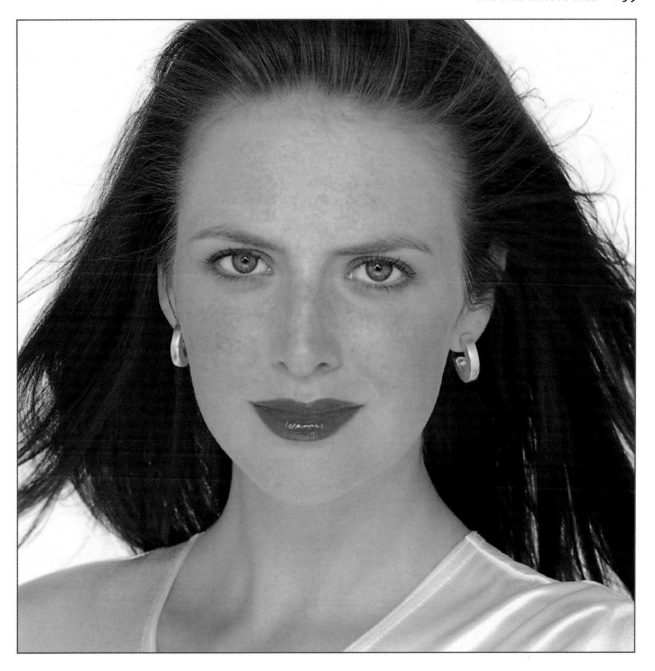

Classic Chic

Whatever your age or colouring, this simple but highly effective classic make-up look will always make a pleasing impact!

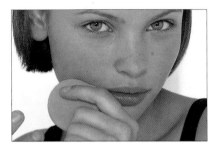

1 Apply a sheer all-in-one foundation-powder. This will give your skin the perfect coverage it needs to carry off strong lips, without clogging up your skin.

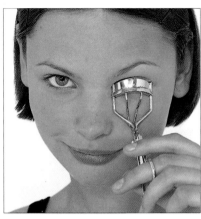

2 The eye make-up for this look is very understated. So, use eyelash curlers to open up your eyes and give them a fresh look.

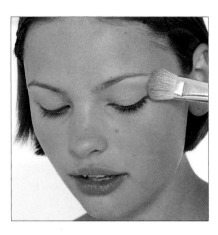

3 Sweep some pale ivory eyeshadow across your entire eyelid using a blender brush. Then complete your eyes with two thin coats of brown-black or black mascara.

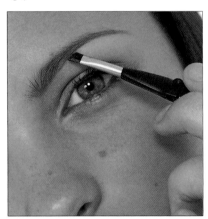

4 Well-groomed eyebrows are essential. Lightly fill in any gaps with a toning eyeshadow. This gives a softer, more natural effect than pencil.

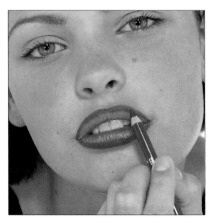

5 Your lips are the focus of this chic look. To ensure that you create a perfect outline, use a toning red lip pencil. Rest your elbow on a hard surface to prevent wobbling.

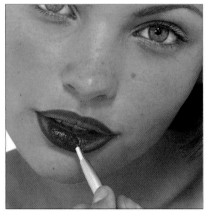

6 Use a lipbrush to fill in with a bold shade of red lipstick. Apply one coat, blot with a tissue, then reapply to help a long-lasting finish.

RED ALERT

Believe it or not, everyone can wear red lipstick. The key to success is to choose just the right shade for your colouring.

Colouring	Choose

Blonde hair, cool skin:
If you're daring enough you can wear any bright red shade. Any bold shade will look really effective and striking on you.

Blonde hair, warm skin:
Lovely pink-reds look wonderful with your colouring. They're delicate enough not to look too harsh, while the pinky undertones complement the warmth of your skin.

Dark hair, cool skin:
Rich blue wine-coloured reds look wonderful on your China doll features. The contrast of dark hair, pale skin and red lips is really stunning!

Dark hair, warm skin:
Rich brick reds and ruby jewel-like shades are very flattering to your complexion, while the intensity of colour looks great against your hair.

Red hair, cool skin:
Choose a delicate orange-red, to add a wonderful splash of colour.

Red hair, warm skin:
Warm, fiery reds with brown undertones, to complement your rich hair colour and rosy skin.

Dark hair, olive skin:
Rich red with orange undertones will flatter your skin. Go for a bold colour, as you can carry it off.

Black hair, brown skin:
Berry reds and burgundy reds look wonderful on your skin.

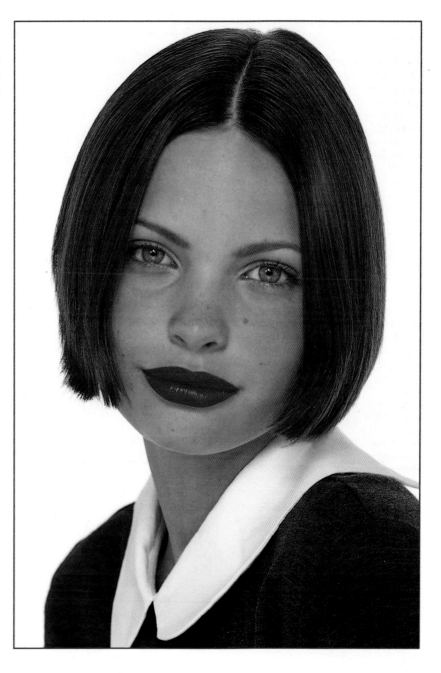

Sunkissed Country Girl

If you want a fresh, outdoor look, try this summery make-up – complete with fake freckles!

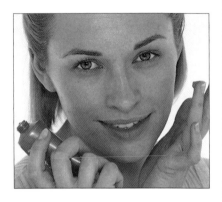

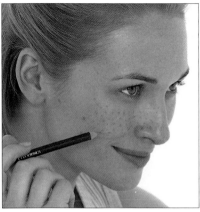

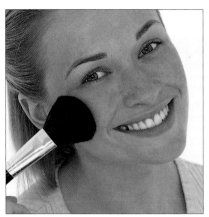

1 You need to avoid heavy foundations when you're outside, so tinted moisturizer is the perfect solution. It'll both nourish your skin and lightly cover any minor blemishes. Apply with your fingertips for ease.

2 If you already have freckles, don't try to hide them – they're perfect for a fresh-air look. If you don't have them, then fake it! Use a mid-brown eyebrow pencil, and dot freckles on the nose and cheeks. Be extra creative, and apply different sizes of freckles for a realistic look.

3 To make your faux freckles look real, soften the edges with a clean cotton bud (swab). Then dust your skin with loose powder to set them in place. A bronzing powder rather than a blusher will give your skin a sunkissed outdoor look. Dust the bronzing powder over your temples, too.

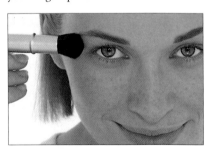

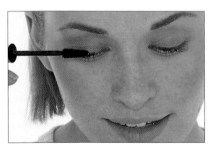

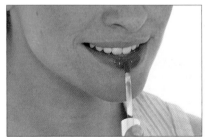

4 Swap to an eyeshadow blending brush to sweep some of the bronzing powder over your eyelids. Natural colours like brown work best for this look. Remove any harsh edges with a clean cotton bud (swab).

5 Keep mascara to a minimum. Choose a natural-looking brown or brown/black shade, and apply just one coat. The waterproof type is great for hot days and sudden downpours, but remember you'll need a waterproof eye make-up remover, too.

6 Don't overpower the look with bold lipstick. Opt for a muted brown-pink shade that's close to your natural lipcolour or use a tinted lipgloss for a natural sheen.

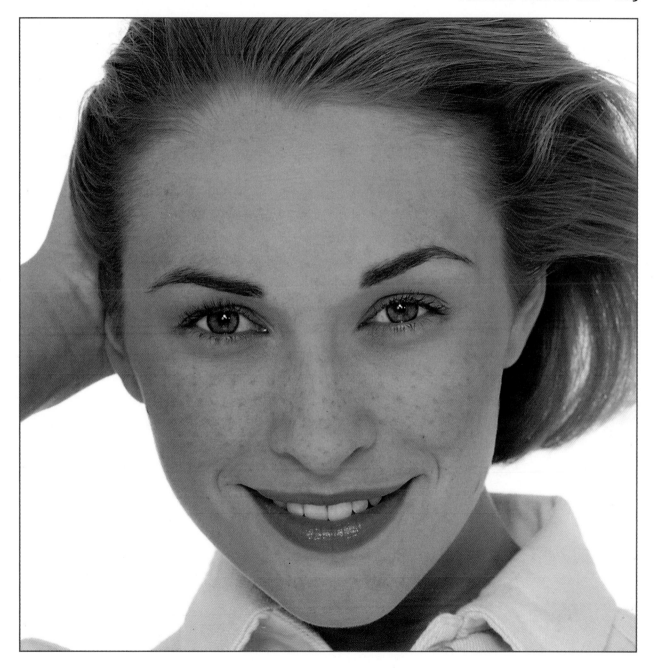

City Chic

Simple, perfectly-applied colours can help you put together a polished image. This stylish, balanced look will make you feel really confident and will leave you ready to get on with the more important things in your day!

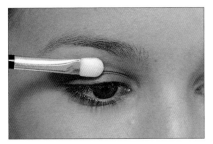

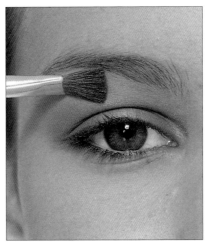

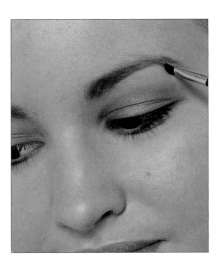

1 After applying a light foundation and dusting your skin with powder to blot out shine, sweep your eyelids with a mid-grey eyeshadow.

2 Use a beige highlighting eyeshadow over your brow bone to soften the edges of the grey shadow. Finish with two coats of mascara.

3 Brush your eyebrows with brown eyeshadow to fill in any gaps. This helps to create a strong frame to your make-up look.

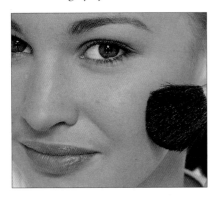

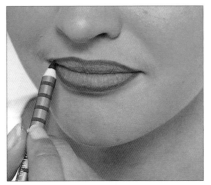

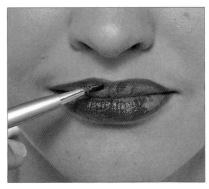

4 A soft pink shade of blusher will give your skin a rosy glow, and co-ordinate the rest of your make-up. And it will give pale work-a-day faces an immediate lift!

5 Use soft blackcurrant lipliner to outline, ensuring you take it well into the outer corners. If you create any wobbly edges, whisk over the top with a clean cotton bud (swab) dipped in a little cleansing lotion. Try again!

6 Fill in your lips with a matching shade of blackcurrant lipstick. Blot your lips with a tissue afterwards for a semi-matte finish that's perfect for a day at the office.

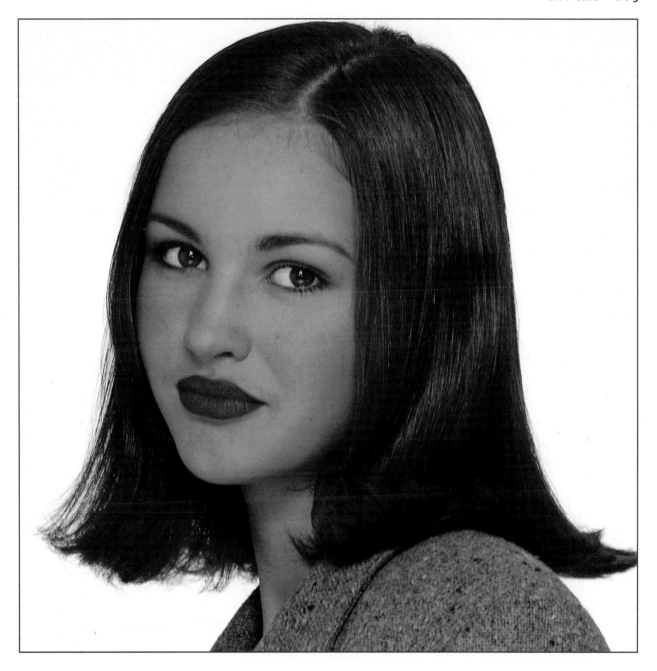

Make-Up To Look Younger!

If you haven't changed your make-up in years, it's a fair bet you're not making the most of your looks. Wearing out-of-fashion make-up is a sure way to add years to your appearance. Our simple make-up rules will help you break out of a beauty rut.

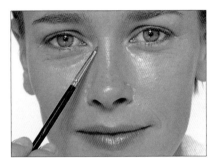

Simple steps to perfect skin

A dull, lifeless skin-tone can make you look, and feel, drab. The great news is, there are now foundations and concealers on the market specially designed to deal with this problem. The formulations contain light-reflective particles, and these bounce light away from your skin. This gives your skin the illusion of added vitality, and helps disguise problem areas such as fine lines and under-eye shadows.

And the good news is that these light-reflective products are not just limited to expensive beauty counters – many more price-conscious companies are now offering them too.

Apply foundation with a damp sponge, blending away harsh edges. This is the stage to apply concealer, dotting it on to under-eye shadows, blemishes and thread veins with a brush. Apply a little at a time, and blend it in thoroughly.

Before you start

Avoid extremes of fashion and bright colours when you're over 40. While younger skins can just about get away with garish make-up, it'll simply emphasize fine lines and wrinkles on most women. Concentrate instead on flattering your looks with subtle colours. So, throw away those traffic-stopping blue eyeshadows and neon lipsticks!

If you haven't a clue where to start, make an appointment for a free makeover at a local beauty counter. This way you'll be able to see which shades suit you before you launch out and buy.

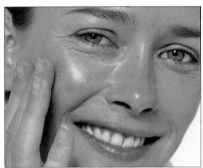

Add a youthful glow with blusher

Forget about adding colour to your skin with foundation – you'll be left with a mask effect and "tidemarks" (streaks) on your jawline. Instead, recreate a youthful bloom with a light touch of blusher. Remember though, to use half as much blusher and twice as much blending as you originally think! The cream variety of blusher is a good one to try, because it will give your skin a soft glow. Dot the blusher onto your skin, and blend with your fingertips.

Lightly set your foundation and blusher with translucent powder. A common mistake among many women is to be heavy-handed with face powder. Applying too much can make it settle into fine lines and wrinkles on your face and emphasize them. Aim for a light touch, which will just blot out shine and set your make-up.

The best way to apply powder is only to blot the areas that need it, then brush away the excess with a large powder brush, stroking the brush downwards to prevent tiny particles catching in the fine hairs on your face.

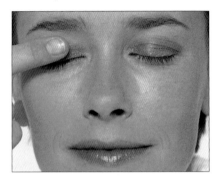

Be subtle with eyeshadow

Many women never perfect the technique of applying eyeshadow. Thankfully, now there's a type of eyeshadow formulation that is a cinch to apply – cream-to-powder eyeshadow. It applies as a smooth cream, and dries quickly to a super-soft powder finish. Opt for a subtle shade, such as mid-brown, grey or taupe.

A good tip if your eyes look rather droopy is to blend eyeshadow upwards and outwards at the outer corners. Always remember to blend it in well.

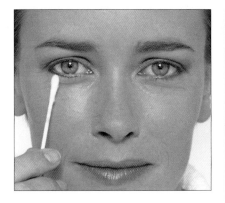

Give eyeliners a miss

Harsh lines of colour close to your eyes can be hard and unflattering. You'll emphasize your eyes much better if you smudge a little neutral-toned powder eyeshadow under your lower lashes with a clean cotton bud (swab).

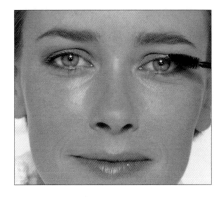

Check your mascara colour

Most women's colouring fades slightly over the years. This means that the black mascara you're used to wearing can now look too obvious and harsh. So, try switching to a lighter shade for a more flattering effect. Apply two thin coats, allowing time for the first to dry thoroughly before you apply the second one.

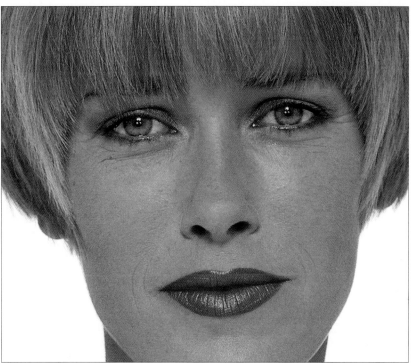

Recreate your lip line

If your lip line has started to fade and your lipstick tends to "bleed" into the lines around your mouth, try using a toning lipliner before you apply lipstick. Check it's firm enough to give a precise line, yet soft enough not to drag your skin. Apply by outlining your top lip first, working from the Cupid's bow outwards to each corner. Then outline your lower lip. Next dust your lips with loose powder to set the lipliner.

Finally, fill in your outline with a moisturizing lipstick. This will also help give a glossy shine to your lips which makes them look fuller. Apply with a lipbrush, blot with a tissue, then reapply for a longer-lasting finish.

Above: Break out of a beauty rut and achieve a youthful new look!

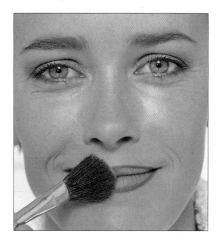

Go For Glamour!

If there's one time you want to make a special effort with your make-up and pull out all the stops, it's a big night out!

We'll show you how to create this stunning look, which combines a mixture of dark and light tones.

Tip
Keep your face free of hair to work!

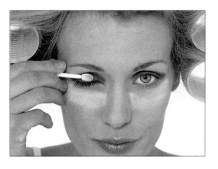

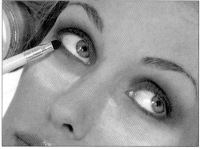

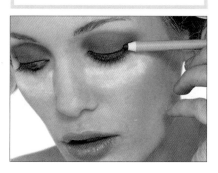

1 After applying your foundation, concealer and powder, you're ready to work on your eye make-up. Sweep a smoky dark brown eyeshadow over your entire eyelid and blend it carefully into the crease. A sponge applicator is easier to use than a brush, but sweep a line of loose powder under your eyes to catch any falling specks of dark shadow.

2 Apply a little of the same shade of eyeshadow under your lower lashes to accentuate the shape of your eyes. This will give a balanced look to your eye make-up and provide a smooth base on which to apply your eyeliner at the next stage. The emphasis for this look is on glamour and impact!

3 Whereas black eyeliner is usually too severe for harsh daylight, it's perfect for this look, which is designed to be seen in softer, sexier light! Using a pencil, carefully draw a fine line above and below your eyelashes. If you find it hard to create a steady hand, try drawing a series of tiny dots, then blend them together with a clean cotton bud (swab).

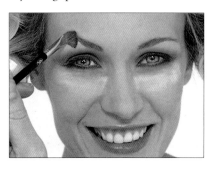

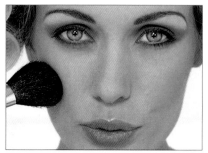

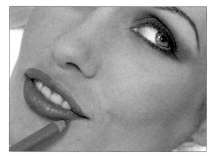

4 To contrast the dark look on your eyelids, sweep a pearlized ivory shadow over your brow bones. Build up the effect gradually. Complete the look with two coats of black mascara.

5 Use tawny blushes or a bronzing powder for this look – they won't compete with the rest of your make-up. Sweep it over your cheekbones and blend away the edges into your hairline.

6 Keeping the lips neutral gives this look its real impact and updates it. Opt for a pinkish-beige shade of lip pencil and smudge it over your entire mouth for a matte, understated effect.

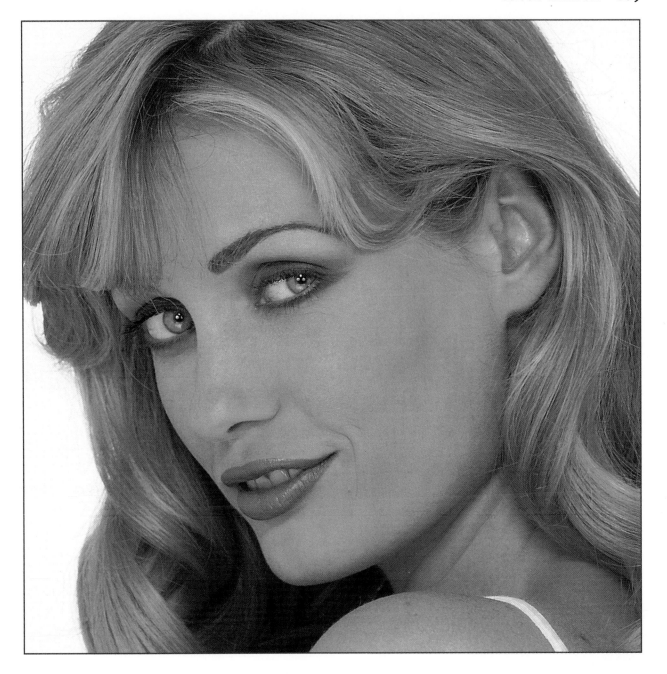

20 Problem Solvers

Whether you have made a beauty mistake, have run out of a vital product or are simply stuck for inspiration on how to make the most of your looks, the following problem solvers are just what you need!

Problem 1
Polish remover has run out
If you want to re-paint your nails, but have run out of remover, try coating one nail at a time with a clear base coat. Leave to dry for a few seconds, then press a tissue over the nail and remove it at once – the base coat and coloured polish will come off in one quick move.

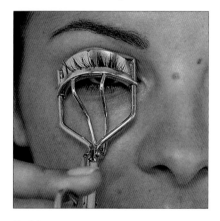

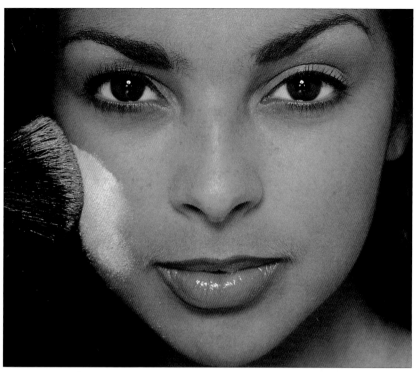

Problem 2
Poker-straight lashes
Do invest in a set of eyelash curlers, as they really make a difference to the way your eyes look. Gently squeeze your lashes between their cushioned pad before applying mascara or you'll risk breaking off the hairs. Curling your lashes makes them look thicker than usual and helps to open up the eyes.

Problem 3
Patchy powder
Provided you apply your powder with a light touch to freshly moisturized skin or on top of foundation that's applied with a clean sponge, it should look perfect. Check your powder is matched closely to your natural skin-tone. So, try dusting a sample of powder onto your skin in natural daylight before buying.

Problem 4
Stained nails
Stained nails are usually caused by wearing dark-coloured nail polish without using a protective clear base coat. Try switching to paler coloured polishes, as these contain lower levels of pigment that are less likely to stain your nails, and use a clear base coat underneath.

Problem 5
Flaky mascara
This usually means the mascara is old and the oils that keep it creamy have dried out. Try not to pump air into the dispenser – go gently when replacing the cap – and replace your mascara every few months. If mascara flakes on your lashes, remove it and make a clean start.

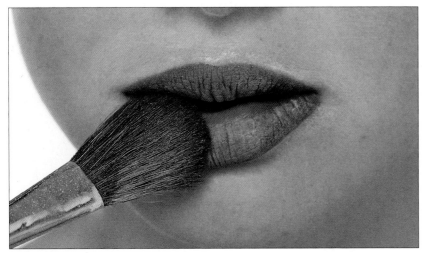

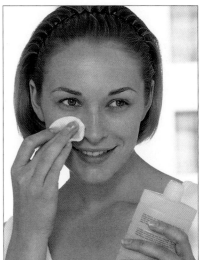

Problem 6
Melting lipstick

If you're out and about and your lipstick is starting to move in the heat, then dust over the top with a little loose powder. This will give it a slightly drier texture, to help it stay put for longer. A little loose powder will also create a lovely matte finish.

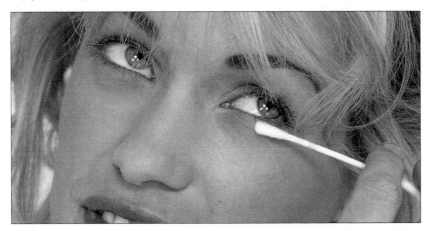

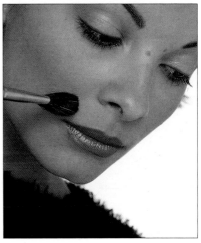

Problem 8
A blemish appears

Start by calming down the blemish by dabbing it with a gentle astringent. Apply a concealer directly onto the blemish or spot, and tidy up the edges with a clean cotton bud (swab). Set in place with a light dusting of loose powder.

Problem 7
Smudged eyeliner

Tidy up the under-eye area by dipping a cotton bud (swab) into some eye make-up remover. Whisk it over the problem area to remove smudges, then re-powder. In future, remember to run a little loose powder over eyeliner to combat smudging.

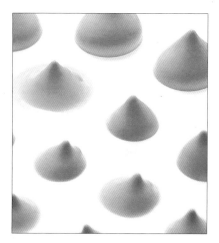

Problem 9
Red-toned skin or embarrassing blushes
A red skin colour can be toned down by smoothing your skin with a specialized green-tinted foundation. Apply with a light touch, just to the areas that really need it. The green pigment in the cream has the effect of cancelling out the red in your skin.

However, to avoid a ghostly glow, you'll need to apply a light coating of your ordinary foundation on top and then set with a dusting of loose powder. This tip is also good for covering the occasional angry spot or blemish.

Problem 10
Flaky lips
If your lips are flaky you'll find it difficult to create a smooth lipstick finish. Slick your lips with petroleum jelly, and leave for 10 minutes to give it time to soften hard flakes of skin. Then cover your index finger with a damp flannel and gently massage your lips. This will remove the petroleum jelly and the flakes of dead skin at the same time.

Problem 11
Bleeding lipstick
Use lipliner to help prevent your lipstick from bleeding into the fine lines around your mouth. Trace the lip outline, then apply lip colour with a brush. Choose a drier textured matte lipstick as they're less prone to bleeding. Also, lightly powder over and around your lips before you start.

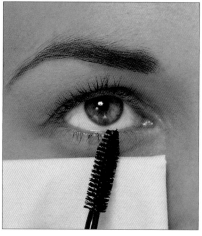

Problem 12
Smudged mascara
If your mascara always seems to run onto your skin, leaving you with "panda eyes", first check that you are using a water-proof variety. Try holding a piece of tissue just underneath your lower lashes while you're applying your mascara to prevent it from getting as far as your skin in the first place.

Alternatively, dip a cotton bud (swab) in eye make-up remover for fast touch-ups before the mascara has a moment to dry on your skin.

To remove excess mascara, place a tissue between your upper and lower lashes and blink two or three times.

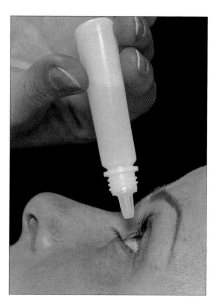

Problem 13
Bloodshot eyes
Red eyes are caused by the swelling of the tiny blood vessels on the eye surface, which can be caused by lack of sleep, excessive time in front of a computer, a smoky atmosphere or an infection. If it's a continual problem, consult your doctor, or ask your optician for an eyesight examination to ensure there's nothing to worry about.

On a temporary basis, you can use eye drops to bring a fresh sparkle back to your eyes.

Problem 14
Tidemarks of foundation
If you find obvious edges to your foundation on your chin, jawline or hairline, blend them away with a damp cosmetic sponge. Do this in natural daylight so you can check the finished effect. Powder as usual afterwards.

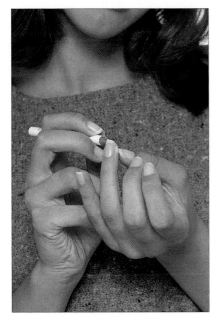

Problem 15
Unhealthy-looking nails
Sometimes, however strong your nails are, their overall effect can be spoilt by yellowing tips. However, you can immediately improve them by running a white manicure pencil underneath the free edges of nail to give them a cleaner appearance. Combine with a coat of clear polish for a fresh, natural nail look.

Problem 16
Yellow teeth
First of all, consult your dentist or dental hygienist for regular check-ups and thorough cleaning. Take heart: yellow teeth tend to be stronger than their whiter counterparts! To make them look whiter, avoid coral or brown-based lipsticks – clear pink or red shades will make your teeth look much whiter in comparison.

Problem 17
Droopy eyes
To help lift the appearance of droopy eyes, sweep a light-toned eyeshadow all over your eyelid. Then apply a little eyeshadow with a clean cotton bud (swab) under your eyes, sweeping it slightly upwards. Apply extra coats of mascara on the lashes just above the iris of the eye to draw attention to the centre of your eye rather than the outer corners.

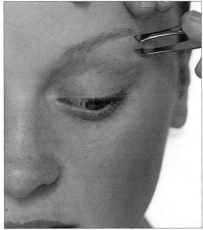

Problem 18
Straggly eyebrows
Tidy them with regular tweezing sessions. The ideal time is after a bath, when your pores will be open from the heat. Before bedtime is also a great idea, so you don't have to face the day with reddened skin!

Quickly brush your brows into place, so you can see the natural shape. Then pluck one hair at a time, in the direction of growth. First remove the hairs between your brows, and then tweeze any stray hairs at the outer sides. As a general rule, don't pluck above the eyebrow area.

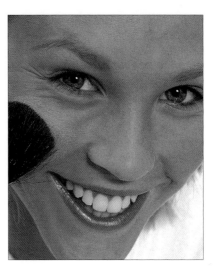

Problem 19
Over-applied blusher
If you've forgotten the golden rule about building up your blusher slowly and gradually, you may need to tone down an over-enthusiastic application of colour. The quickest and easiest way is to dust a little loose powder over the top of the problem area until you've reached a depth of blusher shade that you're happy with.

Problem 20
Over-plucked eyebrows
Choose a natural-looking brown eyeshadow. Then apply it lightly and evenly with a firm-bristled eyebrow brush, using short sharp strokes across the brow. As the hairs that grow back are often unruly, a light coat of clear mascara can be applied to help keep them in place.

Try to ignore the periodic fashions for highly plucked eyebrows. The fashions don't last for long – but eyebrows can take ages to grow back!

50 Fast, Effective Beauty Tips

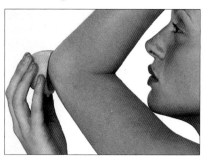

1 Brighten grey elbows by rubbing them with half a fresh lemon – it has a natural bleaching effect. Moisturize the skin afterwards to counteract the drying effects of the juice.

2 Turn foundation into tinted moisturizer by mixing a few drops of it with a little moisturizer on the back of your hand before applying. It's the perfect blend for summer.

3 Carry a spray of mineral water in your handbag to freshen up foundation while you're out and about.

4 Sleeping on your back helps prevent wrinkles, according to recent research. It's certainly worth a try!

5 Dunk feet into a bowl containing warm water and 4 tablespoons of Epsom salts to help ease swollen ankles.

6 If you have very soft nails, file them while the polish is still on to prevent them from cracking.

7 If you find eyebrow tweezing painful, hold an ice cube over the area first to numb the area before you start.

8 Warm up your looks by dusting a little blusher over your temples, chin and the tip of your nose as well as your cheeks.

9 Sweep a little loose powder under your eyes when applying dark shades of eye-shadow to catch any falling specks and prevent them from staining your skin.

10 Make your lips look larger by wearing a bright, light lipstick. Or make them appear smaller by wearing dark or more muted colours.

11 Soak nails in a bowl of olive oil once a week to strengthen them.

12 Keep your smile looking its best by changing your toothbrush as soon as the bristles begin to splay. This means at least every three months. You should brush for at least two minutes, both morning and night.

13 If you don't have a specialized contouring product for your cheeks, simply use an ordinary face powder a couple of shades darker than your usual one to slim round cheeks.

14 Add a drop of witch hazel – available in all good pharmacies – to turn ordinary foundation into a medicated one – it'll work wonders on oily skin or skin which is prone to blemishes.

15 Mascara your lashes before applying false ones to help them stick properly.

16 If you look tired, blend a little concealer just away from the outer corner of your eye – it makes you look as though you had a good night's sleep!

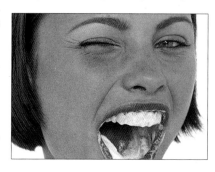

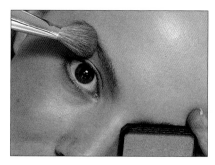

17 Go lightly with powder on wrinkles around the eyes – too much will settle into them and emphasize them.

18 If you haven't got time for a full make-up, but want to look great, paint on a bright red lipstick – it's a happy, glamorous colour which immediately brightens your face.

19 When plucking your eyebrows, coat the hairs you want to remove with concealer – it'll help you visualize exactly the shape of brow you're after.

20 Never apply your make-up before blow-drying your hair – the heat from the dryer can make you perspire and cause your make-up to smudge.

21 The colour of powder eyeshadow can be made to look more intense by dipping your eyeshadow brush in water first.

22 Keep lashes smooth and supple by brushing them with petroleum jelly before going to bed at night, or use to emphasize natural-looking lashes.

23 Apply cream blusher in light downward movements, to prevent it from creasing in specks of colour from catching in the fine hairs on your face.

24 If mascara tends to clog on your lower lashes, try using a small thin brush to paint colour on to individual lashes.

25 Make sure you give moisturizer time to sink in before you start applying your make-up – it'll help your make-up go on more easily.

26 For eyes that really sparkle, try outlining them just inside your eyelashes with a soft white cosmetic pencil.

27 Lip gloss can look sophisticated if you just apply a dot in the centre of your lower lip.

28 Hide cracked or chipped nails under stick-on false ones.

29 If your eyeliner is too hard and drags your skin, hold it next to a light bulb for a few seconds before applying.

30 If you find your lashes clog with mascara, try rolling the brush in a tissue first to blot off the excess, leaving a light, manageable film on the bristles.

31 If you're unsure where to apply blusher, gently pinch your cheeks. If you like the effect, apply blusher in the same area – it'll look wonderfully natural.

32 To prevent lipstick from getting on your teeth, try this tip: after putting it on, put your finger in your mouth, purse your lips and pull it out.

33 Women who wear glasses need to take special advice on make-up. If you're near-sighted, your glasses will make your eyes look smaller. So, opt for brighter,

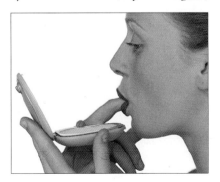

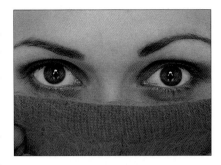

bolder shadows and lots of mascara to ensure they don't disappear. If you're far-sighted, your lenses will make your eyes look bigger and your eye make-up more prominent. So, opt for more muted colours that won't seem so obvious.

34 For a long-lasting blush on sunny days or hot nights, apply both cream and powder blusher. Apply the cream formulation first, set with translucent powder then dust with a little powder blush.

35 Let your nails breathe by leaving a tiny gap at the base of the nail where the cuticle meets the nail – this is where the new nail cells are growing.

36 A little foundation lightly rubbed through your eyebrows and brushed through with an old toothbrush will instantly lighten them.

37 Coloured mascara can look super-effective if applied with a light hand. Start by coating your lashes with two coats of black mascara. Once the lashes are dry, slick a coloured mascara – try blue, violet or green – onto the underside of your upper lashes. Each time you blink your eyelashes will reveal a dash of colour.

38 If you use hypo-allergenic make-up for sensitive skin, remember to choose hypo-allergenic nail polish, too – you constantly touch your face with your hands and can easily trigger a reaction.

39 Make over-prominent eyes appear smaller by applying a wide coat of liquid liner. The thicker the line the smaller your eyes will look.

40 Calm down an angry red blemish by holding an ice cube over it for a few seconds and then apply your usual medicated concealer.

41 If you've run out of loose powder, use a light dusting of unperfumed talcum powder instead.

42 Use a little green eyeshadow on red eyelids to mask the ruddiness.

43 If you've run out of liquid eyeliner, dip a thin brush into your mascara and apply in the same way. It works perfectly.

44 You can dry nail polish quickly by blasting nails with a cold jet of air from your hairdryer.

45 Use a toothpick or dental floss regularly to clean between your teeth, and make sure you visit the dentist every 6 months to avoid serious problems.

46 Apply foundation-powder with a damp sponge for a thicker, more opaque coverage. Applied with a dry sponge, the result will be sheerer.

47 Run your freshly sharpened eyeliner pencil across a tissue before use. This will round off any sharp edges and remove small particles of wood.

48 If you have hard-to-cover under-eye shadows, cover them with a light coat of blue cream eyeshadow before using your ordinary concealer. It really works.

49 Get together with a friend and make each other up – it's amazing how other people picture you – and it's a great way to find yourself a new look.

50 Remove excess mascara by placing a folded paper tissue between your upper and lower lashes and then blinking two or three times.

50 Best Budget Beauty Tips

1 Cotton wool pads (cotton balls) soak up liquids like toner, so dampen them first with water. Squeeze out the excess, then use as usual.

2 A drop of remover added to a bottle of dried-up nail polish will revive it in a few seconds. Shake well to encourage it to mix in thoroughly.

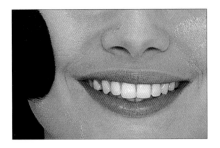

3 Stand a dried-up mascara in a glass of warm water to bring it back to life.

4 Keep new soaps from getting too soft by putting them in a warm cupboard until you need them. This helps dry the moisture out, which makes them harder and longer-lasting.

5 To get the last drop out of almost empty bottles store them upside down overnight. You'll reap the rewards the next morning.

6 Don't rip the cellophane cover off translucent powder – prick a few holes in it instead – it'll stop you spilling and wasting it.

7 Keep perfume strips from magazines in your bag for an instant freshener.

8 Sachets in magazines make ideal travel packs for weekends away.

9 If you've run out of blusher, dot a little pink lipstick on your cheeks and blend well with your fingertips.

10 Look out for "2 for the price of 1" offers on your favourite beauty products. Perhaps split the savings with a friend.

11 Turn ordinary mascara into the lash-lengthening variety by dusting eyelashes with a little translucent powder first.

12 Dust blusher over your eyelids as an instant eyeshadow. It's quick to apply, and will give a balanced look to your make-up.

13 Dab some petroleum jelly around the neck of a new nail polish bottle, and it should be easy to open for the entire life of the product.

14 A cheap way to boost the shine of dark hair is to rinse it with diluted vinegar. Blonde hair benefits from lemon juice. Both act by sealing down the outer cuticles of the hair, helping your hair reflect the light more easily.

15 De-fuzz using a razor with replaceable blades – it works out much cheaper in the end than buying disposable razors.

16 Swap commercial facial scrubs for a handful of oatmeal massaged directly on to your skin – it works really well.

17 Don't use too much toothpaste – it is the brushing action that gets the teeth clean. A pea-sized blob is enough.

18 Pick products in the largest size you can afford – it is much cheaper that way.

19 Don't just shop for beauty goodies in glitzy department stores and fancy pharmacies. Local supermarkets can often offer a surprisingly good range.

20 If you're happy to forgo a fancy label, look out for the great value own-label products at leading drug store chains.

21 Sometimes you're just as well off with cheap alternatives. Opt for those when you can, and indulge yourself with the products that are really worth it.

22 Buy cheap but effective body moisturizers instead of expensive fragranced ones. Then save your money to splash out on your favourite perfume.

23 Now that more companies are offering state-of-the-art products, you can choose affordable products and still get the same results as you would from prestige brands – at a third of the price.

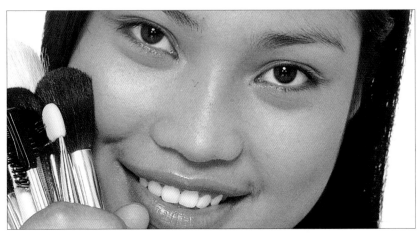

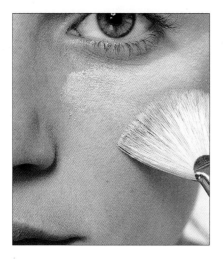

24 Many top make-up, skincare and fragrance companies offer complimentary sample products at their counters. While this is usually at the discretion of the consultant, it is always worth asking, especially if you are already buying something from them.

25 There is a big trend at the moment for 2-in-1 products, and they are always worth trying because they can really save you money. Particularly good buys are shower gels with added moisturizer or body scrubs and shampoos with added conditioner.

26 If you want to indulge in some new make-up but don't know where to start, ask for a makeover at a cosmetic counter. It's the best way to see how colours and formulations look on your skin before buying anything.

27 Store make-up and fragrance in a cool dark place to extend its lifespan.

28 Hair that is all the same length is the easiest and cheapest hairstyle to maintain as it doesn't require as many visits to the hairdresser to keep it looking good.

29 Don't throw away an item of make-up just because the colour is no longer in fashion – it will probably come back again in a few months.

30 Make cheap nail polish last longer by sealing it with a clear top coat.

31 Pure glycerine is an extremely cheap and effective moisturizer when you don't have much to spend.

32 Turn lipstick into lip gloss with a coat of lip balm after applying colour.

33 Double up your lip liner to fill in your lips as well as to outline them.

34 Prise eyeshadows out of their cases, and stick into an old, clean paintbox to create a make-up artist's palette.

35 Add a few drops of your favourite eau de toilette to some olive oil. Use as a scented bath oil as a cheap treat.

36 Neutral make-up colours are a better investment than brighter ones because they look great at any time.

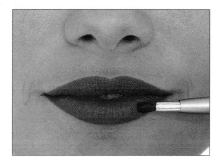

37 Eyeshadow doubles up as eyeliner if applied with a cotton bud (swab). Dampen the end of the bud first for a more dramatic effect.

38 If you are choosing a new fragrance, always buy the weaker and cheaper eau de toilette before splashing out on the stronger and more expensive perfume – in case you change your mind.

39 Check out the model nights at your local hairdressers when trainee hairdressers will style your hair for a fraction of the normal price.

40 Mix different colour lipsticks on the back of your hand with a brush and create a new shade for free!

41 A drop of olive oil rubbed nightly into your nails will help them to grow long and strong, and is much cheaper than shop-bought manicure oils.

42 When you are out of toothpaste, brush your teeth with plain baking soda – it will make them extra white too.

43 To avoid wasting your costly lip and eye pencils, put them in the refrigerator before sharpening to make them less likely to break.

44 Make powder eyeshadows last longer and stay crease-free by dusting eyelids with translucent powder first. It'll absorb the oils from your skin, and keep your make-up looking fresh.

45 Sharpen dull eyebrow tweezers by rubbing sandpaper along the tips.

46 Add a drop of water to the last remains of a foundation to ensure you use every last dot.

47 Keep the plastic seals or paper discs that come with new products. Replace the seals after use to help prevent air from distributing in the make-up and breeding bacteria – which means your product stays fresh until the very end.

48 Spritz your hair lightly with water and re-blow dry to revive products already in the hair, and make your style look as good as new.

49 Add half a cup of bicarbonate of soda (baking soda) to your bath water as a cheap water softener in hard water areas.

50 Use an old clean toothbrush to slick unruly eyebrows into shape.

Your Top 10 Make-up Questions

1 BLUSH BABY

Q: "How can I change the shape of my face using blusher?"

A: To apply blusher, smile, find the apples of your cheeks and dust on the colour above them, blending upwards. For special occasions combine your normal blusher with a barely-there highlighter colour and a shader colour that is slightly darker than your usual blusher to reshape your face. Experiment with the one of following:

■ Slim a round face by sweeping your usual blusher upwards from your cheeks into your hairline. Highlight your cheek-bones, and use shader in the hollows.

■ Soften a square face by concentrating your blusher on the rounded part of your cheeks. Apply shader into the hollows of your cheeks, and also lightly on the square edges of your chin. Dust highlighter on to the bridge of your nose and the tip of your chin.

■ Balance a heart-shaped face by dusting blusher into the hollows of your cheeks. Dust highlighter on to the tip of your chin, and apply shader to your temples, blending it into your hairline.

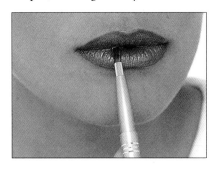

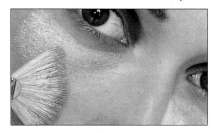

2 24-HOUR LIPSTICK

Q: "Is there any way to make my lipstick stay put all day?"

A: Unfortunately there is no such thing as a 24-hour lipstick, no matter what some cosmetic manufacturers claim! The longest lasting lipsticks are those with the thickest, driest textures, although this can mean they leave your lips feeling quite dry, especially if you use them everyday. Look for lipstick sealers, which are clear gels that you paint over your lips after you've applied your lipstick. Once they're dry, these sealers help your lipstick stay put – at least past your first cup of coffee.

3 OVER-PLUCKED EYEBROWS

Q: "I plucked my eyebrows very thin last year. Now I'd like to grow them back. How can I do it successfully?"

A: Choose a natural-looking brown eyeshadow, then apply it lightly with an eyebrow brush, using short sharp strokes across the brow. The hairs that grow back are often unruly, so apply a coat of clear mascara to keep them in place.

Try to ignore the periodic fashions for highly plucked eyebrows. The fashions don't last long but eyebrows can take ages to grow back! It's better to concentrate on removing stray hairs from beneath the arch and between the brows.

4 COVERING BIRTHMARKS

Q: "Can you recommend something that will cover my birthmark, even when I go swimming?"

A: You need a specialized foundation that will give ultimate coverage, look opaque and be waterproof. Look for a specialized range of camouflage creams tailor-made to cover skin imperfections, such as scars, port wine stains and birthmarks. Their formulation means that they're applied with the fingertips, using a "dab, pat" motion. They are available from specialist make-up suppliers and dermatologists.

5 SPIDER VEINS

Q: "What can I do about the spider veins on my face?"

A: Spider or thread veins, known by their medical name as "telangiectases", are a common beauty problem. An electrologist can treat them for you, by inserting a very fine needle into the vein. The heat from the needle coagulates the blood inside the vein, rendering it inactive. The number of treatments will depend on the number of spider veins you have. In the meantime, cover the veins with a light covering of concealer, applied with a fine brush and set with loose powder.

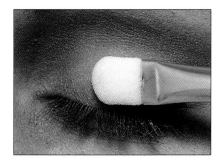

6 MASCARA MATTERS

Q: "My mascara always seems to run on to my skin, leaving me with panda eyes. What can I do?"

A: Choose a waterproof mascara if you are prone to this problem, or "seal" your normal mascara with a coat of clear mascara. Try holding a piece of tissue under your lower lashes while applying your mascara to prevent it getting as far as your skin in the first place.

Alternatively, dip a cotton bud (swab) in eye make-up remover for fast touch-ups before the mascara dries on your skin. A more long-term solution is to regularly have your eyelashes dyed at a reputable beauty salon.

7 COLOUR CODING

Q: "Are there colours which some people can never wear?"

A: As a general rule, everyone can wear every colour. However, if you want to wear a particular colour, you should choose the particular shade of it very carefully. For instance, everyone can wear red lipstick, but in different shades. A pale-skinned blonde will suit a soft pink-red, whereas a warm-toned redhead will be able to carry off an orange-based fiery shade of the colour.

8 SMOOTHER LIPS

Q: "Lipstick always looks awful on my mouth because my lips are so flaky, and it's impossible to create a smooth finish. Is there a solution to this problem?"

A: Slick your lips with petroleum jelly and leave for 10 minutes to give it time to soften hard flakes of skin. Then cover your finger with a damp flannel and massage your lips to remove both the petroleum jelly and the flakes of dead skin.

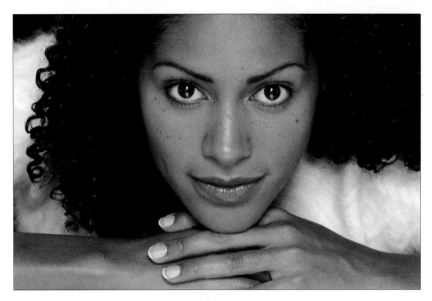

9 PROBLEM POLISH

Q: "I always seem to be left with lots of bottles of nail varnish which I can't use because they're either dried up or full of bubbles, which means they don't go on smoothly. What can I do?"

A: There are some simple solutions to your problem. Dried-up nail polish can be revived by stirring in a few drops of polish remover before using. You can help prevent it from thickening in the first place by storing it in the refrigerator, as the cold temperature will stem any evaporation and thereby prevent any changes in texture.

Bubbles of air in the polish will ruin its finish, as it won't be able to create an even surface. You can prevent this happening by rolling the bottle between the palms of your hands to mix it up before using, rather than shaking it vigorously as this creates the bubbles in the first place.

10 THE CHANGING FACE OF FOUNDATION

Q: "I have difficulty keeping up with the changing colour of my skin in the summer as I gradually get a tan. It's too expensive buying new foundations on an almost weekly basis! What can I do?"

A: None of us can afford to buy new foundation at this rate, and don't despair, because there is really no need. Stick with the colour that suits you when you're at your palest in winter. Then also buy a small tube of dark foundation designed for black skins. Blend just a drop or two into your ordinary foundation on the back of your hand before applying it to your face and blending it in with your tan. This means you can change your foundation daily, without spending a fortune on different shades.

It is worth remembering, too, that foundation works best when it is slightly paler than your natural skin colour.

Fabulous Nail

Your hands say a lot about you. They're one of the first things people notice, because they're constantly on view. As well as using our hands for a wide variety of practical tasks, we use them to help express ourselves and to emphasise what we're saying. That's why it's essential to make the most of yours. Everyone can have great-looking hands and you don't have to have long slender fingers and a perfect set of nails to achieve this.

Some basic care is all it takes to have soft skin and strong, nicely shaped nails. Once you've achieved this, you can experiment with lots of different looks. This book aims to inform and inspire you.

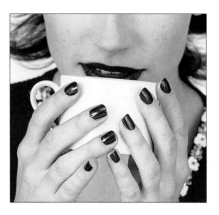

Above: Red nails always look chic and sophisticated.

Right: Try experimenting with different shades of polish.

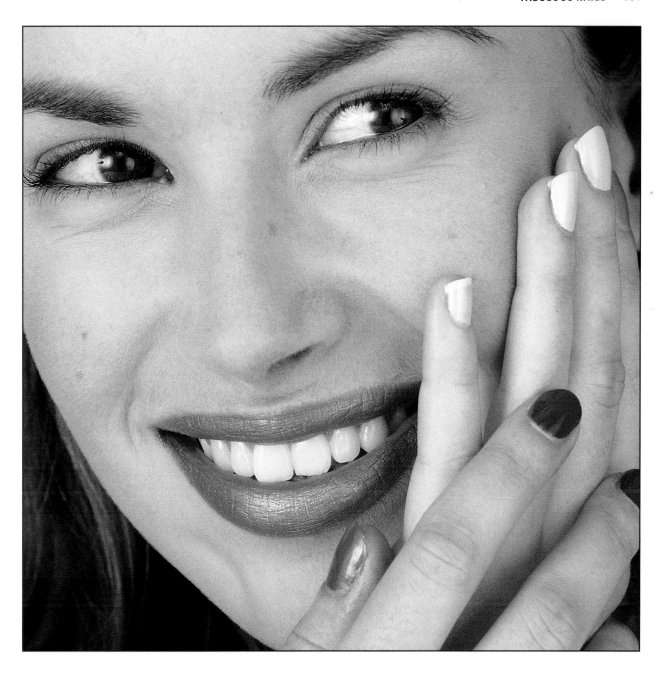

Nail Know-how

Beautiful hands and nails have always been in fashion. In the past very long nails were considered ultra-feminine because it showed that you didn't have to work with your hands for a living. In the 1920s, French fashion designer Coco Chanel sported short nails and showed how attractive they could be. Whatever length your nails are, they'll help you look well groomed if you give them a little care and attention. More than that, you can experiment with different looks to match them to your outfit, express your personality or use them as a striking fashion accessory. The only limit is your imagination.

WHAT IS A NAIL?

A nail is mostly made up from keratin, a protein substance that forms the base of all horny tissue, including your hair. It's whitish and translucent in appearance and allows the pinkish colour of the nail bed underneath to be seen. A nail doesn't contain any nerves or blood vessels. The purpose of nails is to protect your fingers, so you can do a wide variety of tasks.

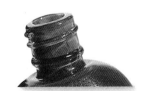

Above: Try a classic red manicure.

Nail bed

The part of the skin the nail rests on. It has many blood vessels that provide the nourishment the nail needs to grow.

Nail root

This is at the base of the nail and is attached to an actively growing tissue known as the matrix.

Free edge

The part of the nail that reaches over the top of the fingertip.

Nail body

The visible portion of the nail that sits on top of the nail bed and extends from the root to the free edge. It is made of lots of thin layers that are held together by oil and moisture to keep it resilient.

Matrix

The part of the nail bed that lies beneath the nail root. It contains nerves, lymph and blood vessels to nourish the nail and produces new cells that create and harden the nail. The matrix will continue to grow as long as it receives nutrition and isn't damaged by injury.

Lunula

The "half moon" located at the base of the nail. The light colour of the lunula is caused by the reflection of light where the matrix and the connective tissue of the nail bed join.

Cuticle

The thin strip of skin around the base of the nail that protects the new cells underneath from infection or damage.

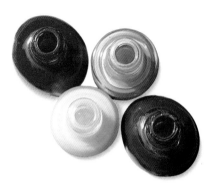

Above: Be as conventional, or as outrageous, as you like when it comes to nail polish colour.

DID YOU KNOW?

■ On average, nails grow about 3 mm (1/4 inch) a month.

■ Nails grow faster in summer time than in the winter.

■ Nails also grow at a faster rate during pregnancy.

■ If you lose a nail owing to an accident, it will take about six months to grow back.

■ Your middle fingernail grows the quickest while the thumbnail grows the slowest.

■ Your toenails grow more slowly than your fingernails.

Right: The natural look can also show off well manicured nails.

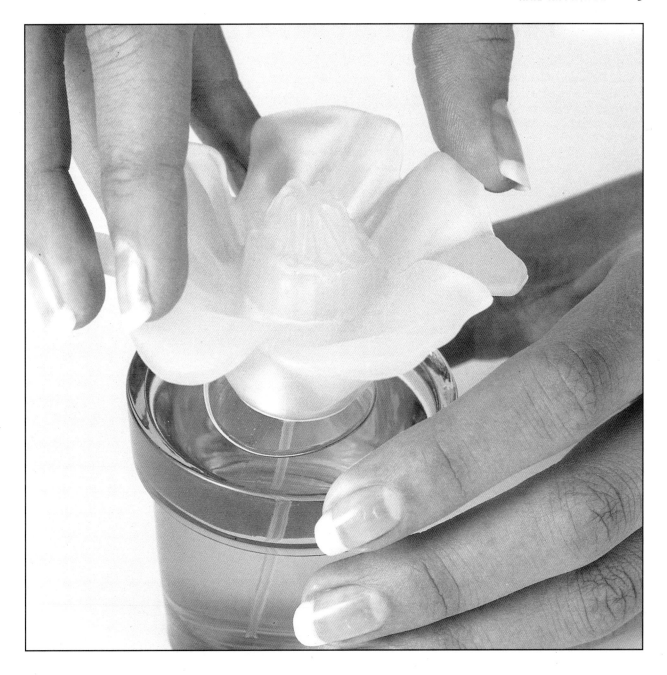

The Essential Manicure Kit

If you're serious about having beautiful nails, you need the right tools for the job. While you don't have to have tray upon tray of equipment like they do in beauty salons, you do need these essential items:

Nail files

Emery boards are the best type to choose, and they come in different levels of coarseness. For most people, a medium grade emery board is very useful for shortening nails, and a fine grade one is good for finishing nails and smoothing away any snags. Replace them regularly, as use soon wears away the edges.

Nail buffer

These come in all shapes and sizes. They usually combine three buffing surfaces to smooth away ridges from the surface of your nails and give a wonderful shine. Try to buy a slim one as they're much easier to use.

Manicure scissors

These are useful when you want to trim long nails without spending a long time wielding a nail file. However, always buff any rough edges from your nails after using scissors.

Manicure bath

This is an instant way to bring a touch of the beauty salon into your own nails.

Right: Face up to beautiful nails.

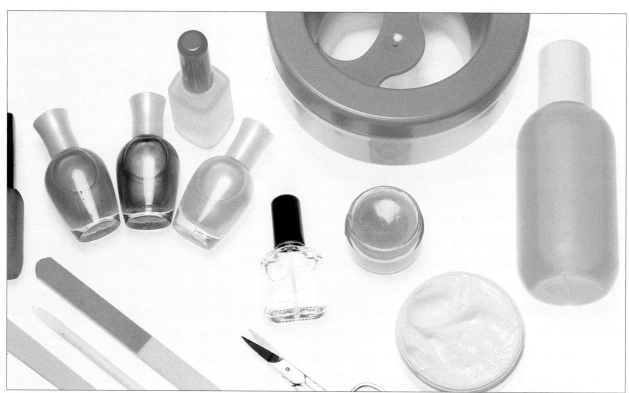

Above: The perfect manicure kit. Clockwise from left: nail file; hoof stick; buffer; polishes; base coat; manicure bath; polish remover; hand cream; treatment oil; manicure scissors; top coat.

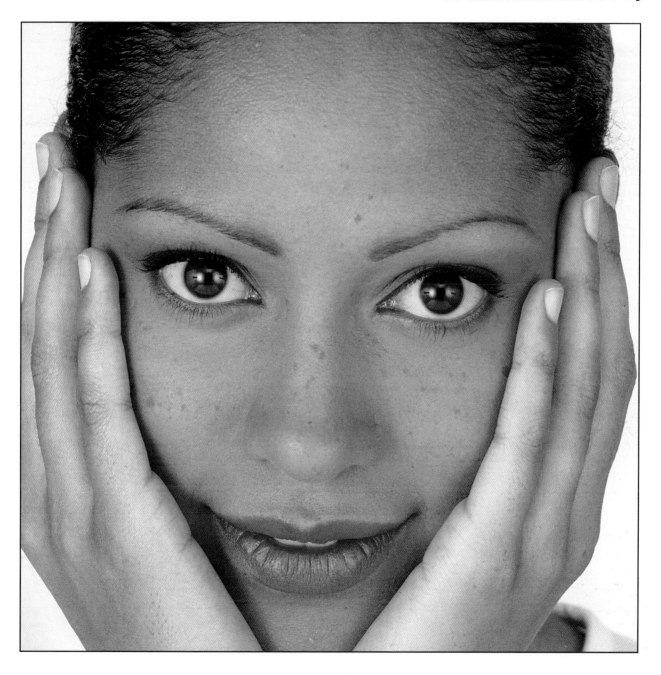

Manicure baths are good for holding cleansing ingredients for use on your nails. The top is shaped so you can place your nails into the liquid without spilling it. However, there's no need to buy a specialist manicure bath – any small, shallow bowl will be just as effective.

Hoof stick

These wooden sticks have a rubber tip on the end, shaped like a horse's hoof, to help you push back the cuticles. The other end can be used to gently scrape away any material from beneath the nails.

Cuticle softeners

These soften cuticles, making it easier to push them back. They're also useful for helping to loosen any stubborn skin that's stuck to the nail bed. Cuticle softeners are available in various formulations – from clear liquids you paint on, to thick creams you massage into the cuticle.

Hand cream

This is essential for helping to seal moisture into the skin on your hands. The oils in the formulation also help to strengthen weak nails. Available as lotions and creams – the drier your skin, the richer the formulation you should choose.

Nail treatment oil

Special treatment for weak or fragile nails. Apply it on a daily basis and you'll soon reap the benefits.

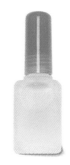

Above: Apply base coat to bare nails before coloured polish.

Base coat

This is applied to bare nails and will help create a smooth surface before you apply coloured polish.

Coloured polishes

It's up to you how many you choose, but a wardrobe of colours will allow you to match your manicure to your outfit.

Clear top coat

This is applied over dry nail polish. It lengthens the lifespan of coloured polish because it helps prevent chipping.

Polish remover

This contains solvents to dissolve old nail polish. Look for acetone-free varieties as they're more gentle on your nails.

Left: Build up a wardrobe of polish colours so you can really express yourself!

Right: A simple glass bowl from the kitchen cupboard will double up as a manicure bath.

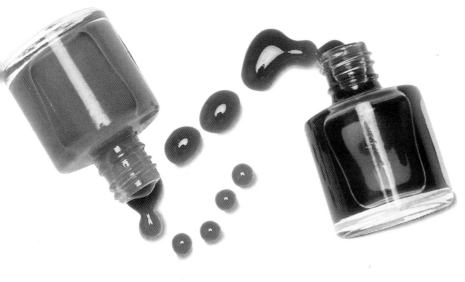

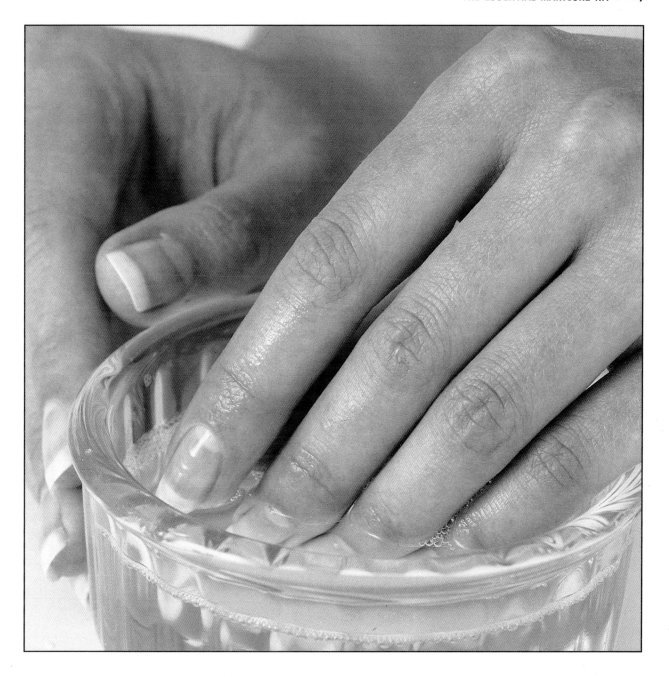

Hard as Nails!

Weak, flaky nails are the most common manicure complaint. While there's no single magic formula to transform fragile nails into tough talons, there are lots of things you can do to help yourself grow long, strong, beautiful nails. Here are some of the best suggestions.

TOP 10 TIPS TO STRENGTHEN NAILS

1 Always wear rubber gloves when washing up the dishes – soaking nails in water is the number one enemy against nail strength. Also, the detergents will strip away the oils your nails need to be strong. If you find that moisture levels build up in the gloves as your hands perspire, wear a pair of thin cotton gloves underneath to absorb the moisture and protect your nails. Healthier nails are stronger nails.

2 Hand models always wear gloves for household or gardening chores. The chemicals in cleaning materials won't do your hands or nails any good and gardening is sure to leave you with damaged nails.

3 Look for nail polish removers that are acetone-free. This ingredient can leave your nails very dry, which means they're more liable to break. Most good handcare ranges offer them.

4 Don't use your nails as a tool. Even the healthiest, strongest set of nails won't stand up to being used as levers or scrapers. Remember to take a moment to find the right tool for the job rather than risk having to grow your nails from scratch again.

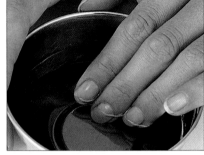

Above: Simple and effective. Pure olive oil will strengthen weak or fragile nails.

5 Soak your bare nails in a bowl of olive oil. Leave them there for 10 minutes, then wipe away the excess with some cotton wool (cotton balls).

6 Most good nailcare ranges offer a nail strengthener lotion to help prevent weak nails from splitting or breaking. Apply it under your base coat.

7 Use the finishing side of a nail buffer to stimulate the circulation of blood in the nail bed.

8 Apply hand cream after each time you wash your hands because it'll help build up oil levels in your nails. Take the time to rub a little into each nail.

9 Once a week, apply a layer of intensive hand cream before bed. Then pull on a pair of white cotton gloves – most good chemists sell them. This will allow the creams to penetrate your hands and nails, and you will wake up to stronger nails.

10 Keep your nails at a sensible short length – they'll be less liable to break.

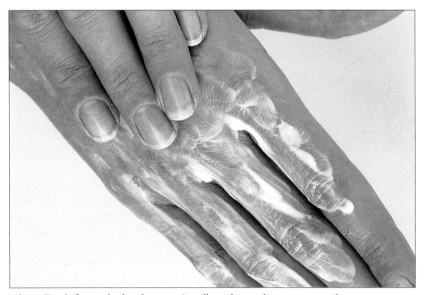

Above: Don't forget the hand cream. It will work wonders on your nails, too.

Right: Toughen up your act for longer, stronger nails.

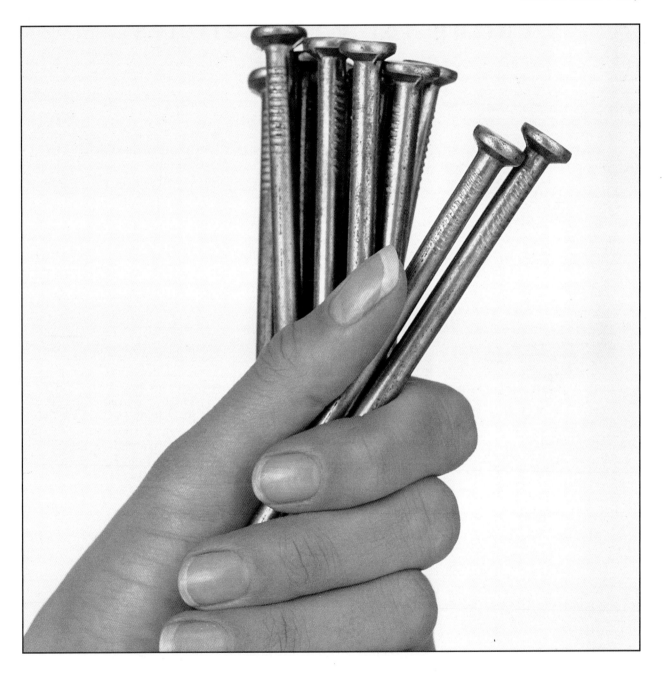

Caring for your Cuticles

Look at any beautiful pair of hands, and you'll see cuticles that are neat and well cared for. Ensuring that your cuticles are well cared for is the cornerstone of any manicure regime.

WHAT IS A CUTICLE?

The thin strip of skin that runs along the base of the nail is called a cuticle. It protects the nail by acting as a barrier against any bacteria that may try to work their way under the nail and damage the live cells that are being formed just underneath.

Cuticle care

It is very important to care for your cuticles properly. If they're neglected and become dry, you could be left with sore, infected nails. If they're pushed back roughly, you run the risk of damaging the new cells underneath. What's more, rough, overgrown cuticles make your hands appear uncared for. A little regular care will ensure that your cuticles are healthy and neat.

CUTICLE TREATMENTS

■ The best time to push back dry or ragged cuticles is right after a bath. You'll get a neater result and find any pieces of skin that adhere to the nail bed easier to remove.

■ Never use clippers on your cuticles. You'll risk leaving your fingers sore and open up your nails to infection. (Many manicurists won't use them for this reason.) Also, using clippers on your cuticles can make them become tougher and thicker than before.

■ There are many cuticle softening creams on the market that help soften the cuticle to make it easier to push back. Modern formulations are fast-acting – that is, you only have to wait a few minutes for results.

■ Nail oils are good news for cuticles. As well as strengthening the nail, they also soften and condition dry cuticles. If you don't have any specialist oil, ordinary olive oil or baby oil will do the trick. Apply it on a daily basis.

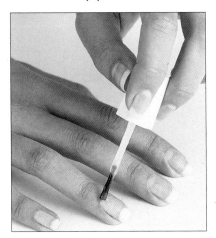

1 Apply a little cuticle softener to the cuticle on each nail. Massage it well into the base of the nail with your fingers to ensure that it works properly.

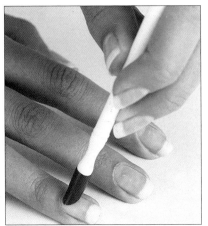

2 Leave it to work for three minutes, or as long as instructed. Then gently push your cuticles back using a hoof stick. If you don't have a hoof stick, use a cottonbud (swab).

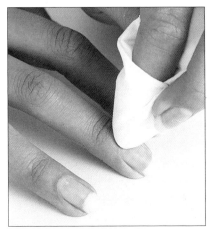

3 Remove any residue with a tissue. Rinse your nails in warm water to ensure that your nails are really clean.

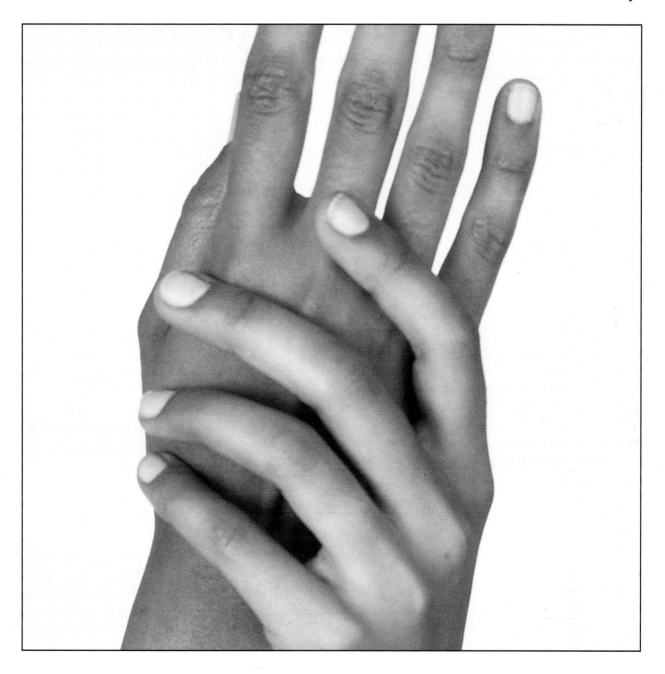

Filing your Nails

It is worth learning the proper filing techniques so you can shape your nails without damaging them.

FILE STYLE

■ While steel nail files may last a lifetime, they're a bad choice because they can tear or split your nails. It's much better to buy a packet of emery boards instead. A general rule to follow is, the weaker your nails are, the finer the emery board you should choose.

■ Have a few nail files on the go at a time. Carry one in your bag or purse at all times, so you can smooth a nail if it snags – rather than having to sacrifice the whole nail tip because it tears.

■ Don't file nails when they're wet because they are more liable to break. If you have extremely weak nails it may be a good idea to file them into shape while you're wearing nail polish for added protection.

■ Never file backwards and then forwards as this can cause the nail layers to split. File in one direction only, using the smooth side of an emery board. Hold the emery board under the nail at a 45 degree angle.

■ Don't file deeply down into the sides of your nails because it exposes the underlying sensitive skin and can lead to infection. It also dramatically weakens your nails.

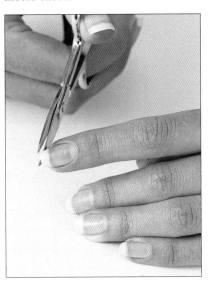

1 If you're making long nails quite a bit shorter, it's quicker and more practical to trim off the excess with a pair of nail scissors. Cut from the side to the middle of the nail, to the length you want. Then repeat on the other side. Don't worry about the final shape at this stage, as you'll correct any defects with the nail file.

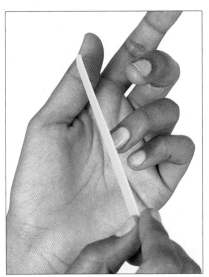

2 File each nail from the side to the centre, holding the emery board at a 45 degree angle. This tilting will ensure that you mainly file the underside of the nail. Repeat on all the nails.

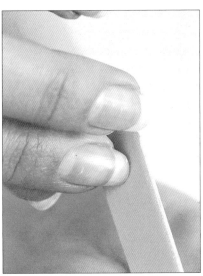

3 Hold the file vertically to file just the tip of the nail using a downward motion.

WHAT SHAPE SHOULD I CHOOSE?

Nails vary greatly in shape, but most usually fall into one of four types – square, round, oval and pointed.

■ Nails can be filed in a variety of ways. A slightly squared oval is the most natural looking and flattering shape for all nails. It's also a nail saver because you don't need to file too deeply into the sides of the nails – this is where most breakages start.

■ If you're not sure what shape to file your nails, look at the shape of your nail at the base. The tips of your nails look good when they mirror this shape.

■ Don't wear your nails ridiculously long – it's impractical and old fashioned. Turn your palms facing you. If you can't see any nails extending over your fingertips then your nails are too short. You should see about 1/2cm (1/4 inch) of nail tip for the ideal length.

■ If you work with your hands, a shorter, more rounded shape is usually better in order to avoid nail breakage.

■ If your nails are thin or weak, it's best to keep them fairly short – or they're sure to break. Shorter nails also means stronger nails.

Right: Beautifully shaped nails can easily carry off the brightest and boldest shades of polish.

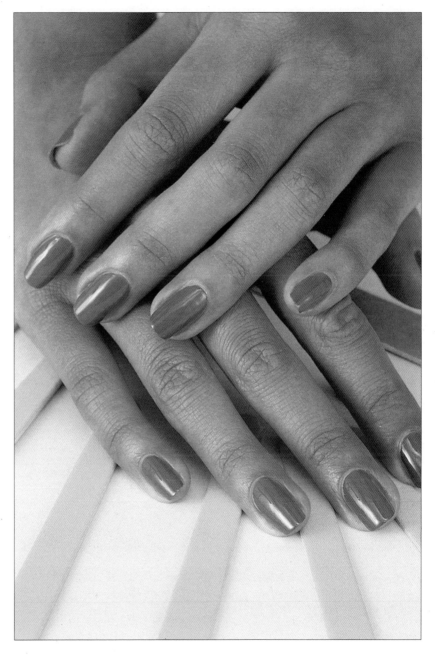

Pretty Nails, No Polish

Use a nail buffer to create a look that requires low maintenance, is as shiny as clear polish and lasts for up to a week. The only tool you need is a buffer: use the pink side to prime your nails, the white to smooth ridges and the grey to add shine.

THE BENEFITS OF BUFFING

■ Buffing won't dry out or damage your nails as polish can.

■ It's an excellent way of boosting the circulation of blood in the nail bed, which means healthier, stronger nails in the long term.

■ It will make all nails look better because it smoothes out tiny imperfections in the surface, helping to make them shine.

■ It's a natural look that goes with any make-up look.

■ It's quick and easy, as there is no waiting for polish to dry.

■ It's an easy technique that anyone can master! If you haven't tried many manicure techniques before, it's a good place to start!

> **Tip**
> Don't buff until you get a burning sensation at your fingertips – it's a sign you're overdoing it and wearing down the nail.

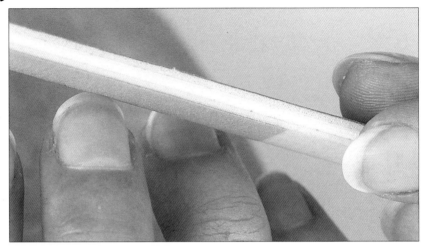

1 Wash your hands with soap and water and dry them well so your nails are free from surface oils. Then, using the rough pink side of the buffer, gently buff backwards and forwards, working from the base of your nails to the tips. This temporarily roughs up the surface of your nails.

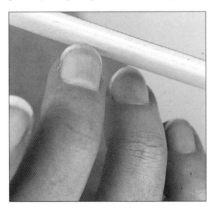

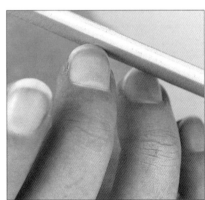

2 Switch to the soft white side of the buffer and buff again. Use a very light pressure and keep going until your nails look nice and shiny.

3 Finish by using the same motion with the smooth grey side until your nails really gleam. A couple of minutes spent at this stage will achieve a shine that lasts for a long time.

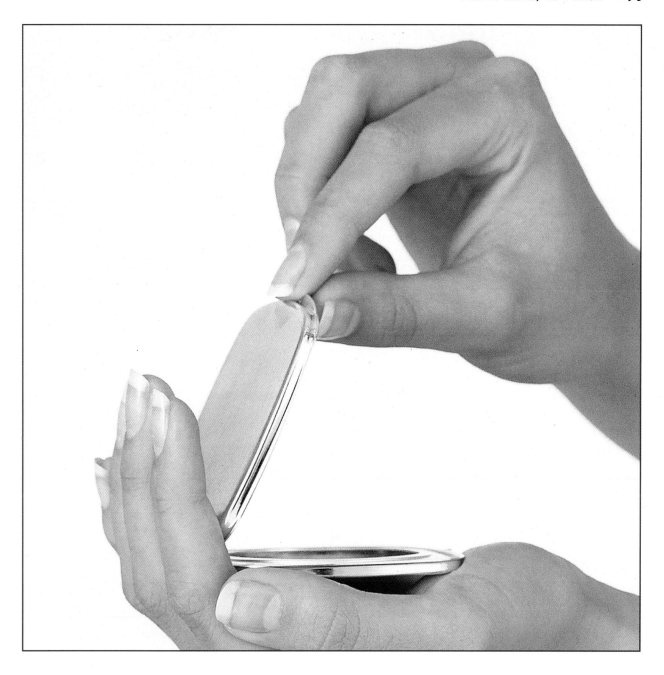

Clean, Simple Nails

Everyone loves nails that look healthy and well cared for. Accentuate the tip with a sweep of white nail pencil, then add instant shine with a coat of clear polish. It couldn't be simpler!

ALL WHITE ON THE NIGHT

A white nail pencil is a great manicure tool to keep on hand. Even if you've managed to grow your nails to a respectable length, the tips may not look as even and white as you would like. An instant solution is to apply a little white nail pencil under the free edges of your nails. It lasts until the next time you wash your hands.

■ If you don't have an ordinary clear polish to hand, then a base coat or top coat will work just as well.

■ You can use white eyeliner pencil instead, if you prefer.

■ Sharpen the pencil before using it to make it hygienic to use.

■ If the white pigment clumps under the nail, sweep over it with a clean cotton-bud (swab).

> **Tip**
> Keep the pencil well sharpened to make it easier to apply. If it is quite soft, try storing it in the refrigerator between uses.

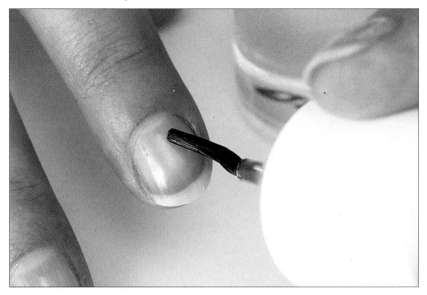

1 Apply a coat of clear polish. Allow it to dry thoroughly before applying a second coat. Two thin coats give a better finish than one thick coat.

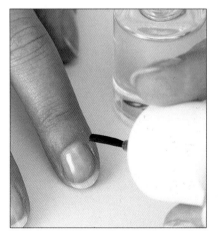

2 Apply a second coat to build up a tough, glassy sheen.

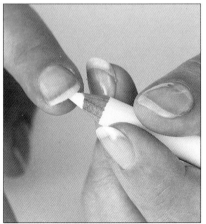

3 Run the white pencil under the free edges of your nails.

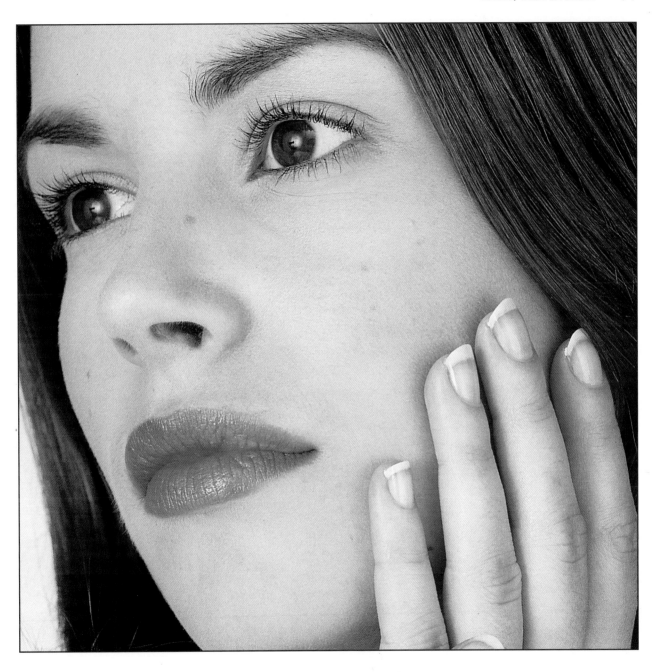

The Classic Red Manicure

Red nails always look chic and sophisticated, whether you want to look stylish by day or sexy by night. What you need is a steady hand and a little time to achieve a look that never goes out of fashion.

THE RIGHT RED FOR YOU

Just take a look at the cosmetic counters and you'll discover that there are literally dozens of different reds to choose from. For instance, a soft strawberry red is worlds apart from a striking pillarbox (cherry) shade of red. A good way of deciding which shade of red is right for you is to take a look at the tone of the skin on your fingers – it will suit some shades of red better than others.

■ Pale skin – crimson will create a dramatic contrast against your skin tone.

■ Freckled skin – orange reds will look striking without overpowering your skin.

■ Warm skin – pinky reds will enhance the warm tones of your skin without being too harsh.

■ Olive skin – fiery reds with brown undertones will flatter your skin.

■ Black skin can carry off berry red or burgundy.

Tip

If you have long, elegant fingers, you can carry off dramatic deep reds, russets and burgundies with style.

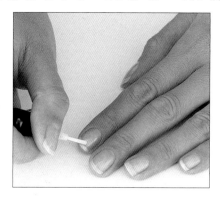

1 Start with the little finger on your right hand and work inwards, then do the same for your left hand. First apply a coat of clear base coat to prevent the red pigment in your nail polish staining your nails.

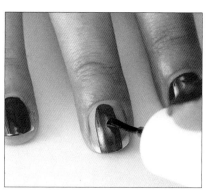

2 Apply a stripe of red polish down the centre of your nail.

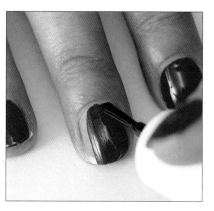

3 Paint a strip of colour along the side of each nail to finish. The side strokes should meet with and overlap the centre one. Don't overload the brush – one dip into the bottle should do an entire nail. Wait until the colour dries, then apply another coat.

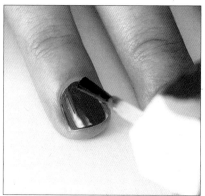

4 Finish with a coat of clear top coat to help guard against chipping.

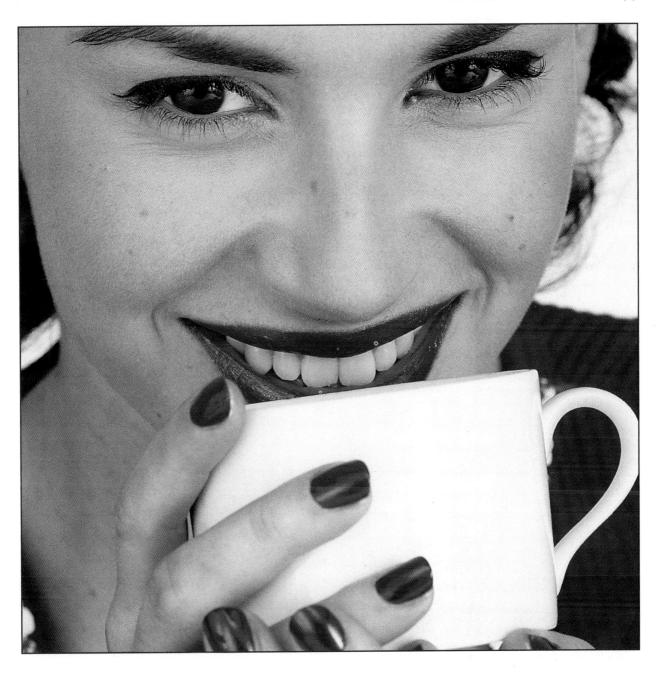

The 1950s Manicure

In the 1950s, many women wore another version of the classic red manicure. This was basically the same look, except that the half moons at the base of each nail were left clear. This look has come back into fashion recently because it looks so good, but you need a steady hand to apply it.

MANICURE TIPS

■ This is a difficult look to achieve well. If you find the brush is quite unwieldy, pull out a few bristles to make a slimmer brush that's easier to handle.

■ This look suits long slim nails the best. If you have very wide nails, it is best to avoid this look as it'll simply accentuate the breadth of your nails.

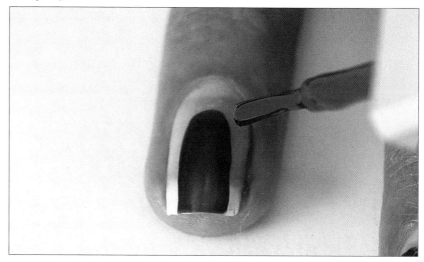

1 Over a clear, protective base coat, apply a stripe of red nail polish down the centre of the nail, starting just above the moon at the base of your nail.

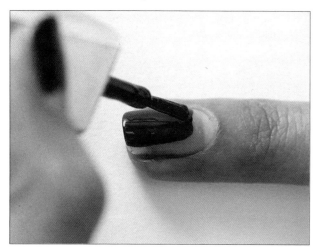

2 Apply a strip of colour to each side of the nail, following the line of the half moon.

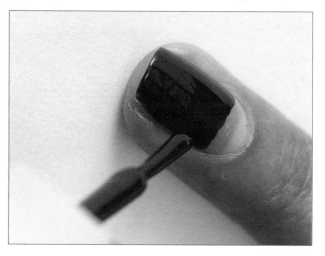

3 Wait until it is completely dry, then apply a second coat of nail polish. Finish with clear top coat, applied over the whole of the nail.

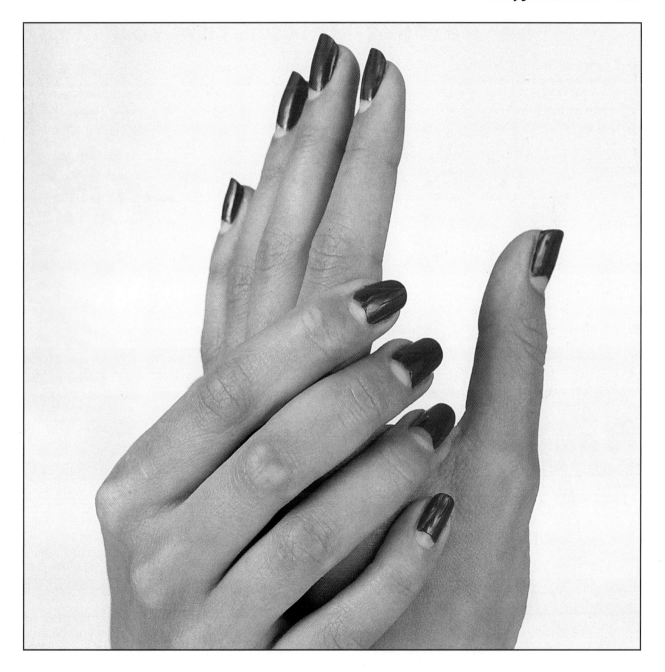

The Perfect Polish for You

There's a vast range of nail polish colours on the market. Experiment to find your favourites, but first take a few factors into account when choosing the most popular nail polish colours.

■ Pale beiges and ivories are a very good choice for short nails because they create a "barely there" finish. They are also a good choice if you don't have much time for manicures, because they don't show up chips quite as much as other colours.

■ Corals, oranges and purples look fabulous against tanned, olive or dark skins. However, avoid them if you have nicotine-stained fingers as they'll just emphasise the problem.

■ Red is a wonderful bold colour on all skin tones and nail lengths. As a general rule, the longer your nail, the brighter the red you can carry off. However, red only looks good on well-cared for hands. There's nothing worse than red, bitten nails!

■ Soft pinks suit everyone's skin tone. Also, they don't require perfect nails to look good.

■ Browns and burgundies work best on young, slim hands. They can emphasize large knuckles or lines.

Below: New nail polish colours are always fun to try – your colour choices are endless.

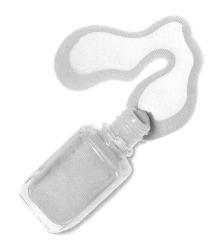

Above: A soft pink polish will complement most people's skin tone.

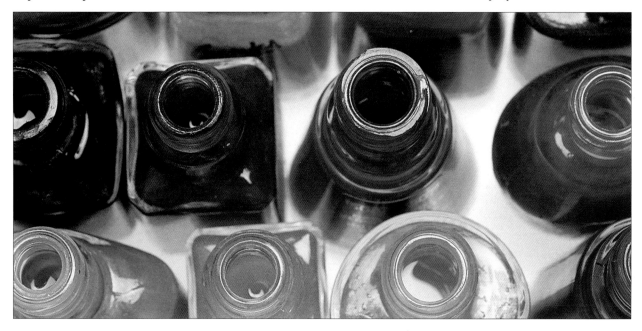

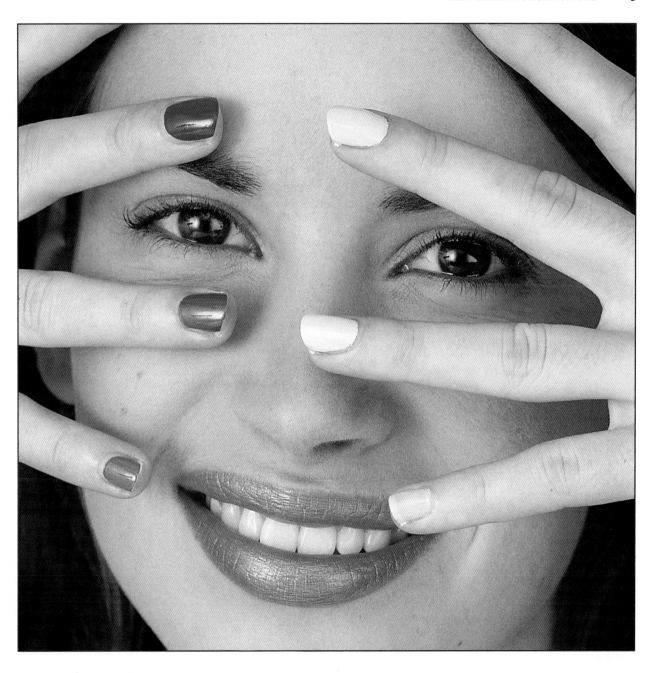

The French Manicure

The French manicure is a look that everyone loves because it makes all lengths of nails look clean and healthy. It combines a pink polish over the entire nail with white tips. It's suitable for all occasions, from an ultra-natural to a bridal look. It does take a little practice to get right at first, but it's worth persevering.

Getting the look right

Most ranges of polish include soft pink and white shades that enable you to create the French manicure look. However, it's also worth looking out for special kits that contain everything you need to get the look right. Some kits come complete with pieces of tape that you lay across the nail to allow you to paint on the white polish. However, these tend to leave a ridge of polish when they're removed, which can ruin the look. It's better to draw the white tips freehand. Use a small paintbrush if you find that the brush supplied is too unwieldy.

The American manicure

Another lovely, but less well known manicure look is the American manicure. It's similar to the French manicure, except that you replace the pink base polish with a creamy buff or beige shade. You may find that it's more flattering to your skin tone than the pink polish.

> ### Tip
> The key to this look is to wait for each coat to dry thoroughly before applying the next – otherwise, you're sure to end up with smudges.

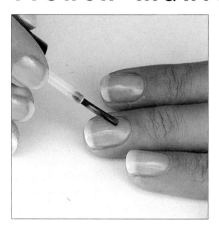

1 Apply a clear base coat to protect your nails and help to prevent chipping.

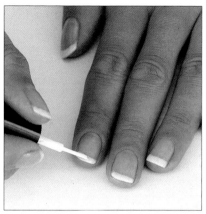

2 Apply two thin coats of white polish to the tips of your nails. Try to apply it in one long stroke, working from one side of your nail to the other.

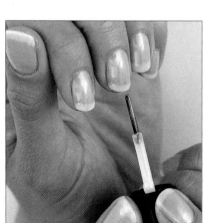

3 Allow the white polish to completely dry, then apply a coat of pink polish over the entire nail. If you like a very natural finish, just apply one coat of pink polish; if you prefer a bolder effect, apply two coats.

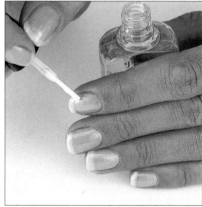

4 Apply a clear top coat over the entire nail for added protection.

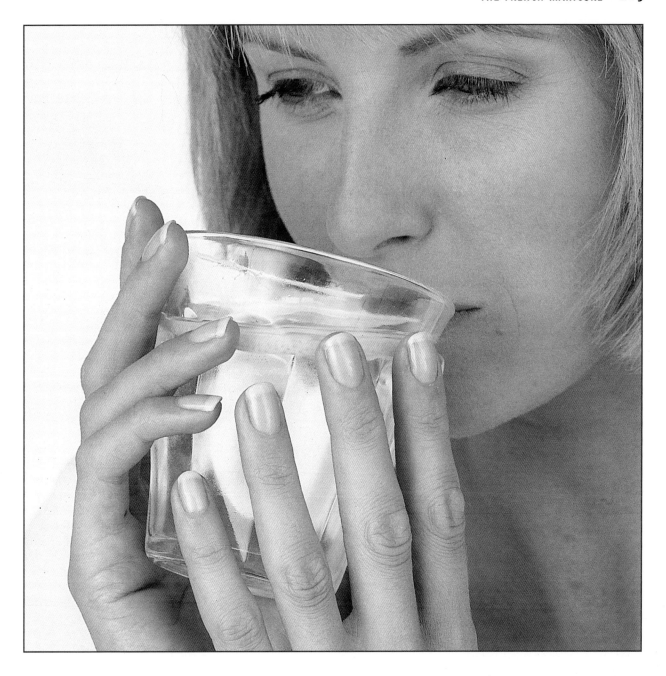

Pearly Polish

Even the shortest nails look great with a coat or two of polish that has a shimmering, pearlized finish. It's a soft, pretty look that suits everyone. Because it creates quite a subtle finish, you can wear it with any make-up look. Pearlized nail polish gives an especially pretty look in the summer and for holidays because the shiny particles glisten in the sunshine.

■ Pearly nail polish tends to give quite a sheer finish. Apply only one coat for a pretty, "barely there" effect.

■ Pearlized polish tends to chip more easily than other types, so be prepared to remove it after a couple of days. However, you can enhance its life by applying two coats of clear polish over the top to seal in the effect.

■ Originally, pearly polish was only available in a creamy mother-of-pearl finish, but today there are also purples, pinks and corals to choose from.

■ Some women with delicate skin find they're particularly sensitive to pearlized polish, so take care. Look for the hypo-allergenic variety.

Right: Build up the coats to intensify the finished result.

Right: Shimmering mother-of-pearl nails look good on everyone.

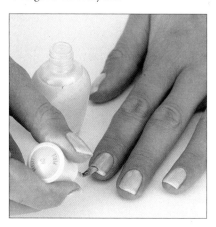

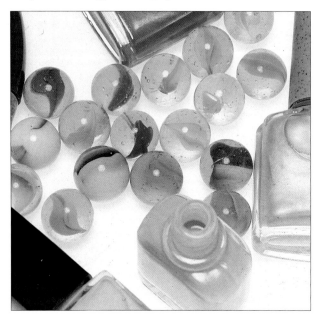

Above: Keep your nail polish colours subtle with pretty shades of pink and plum.

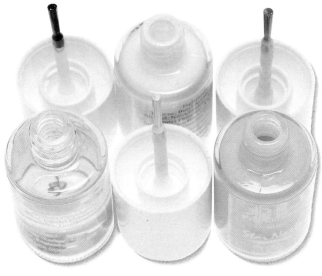

Above: Add a hint of shimmer to your nails.

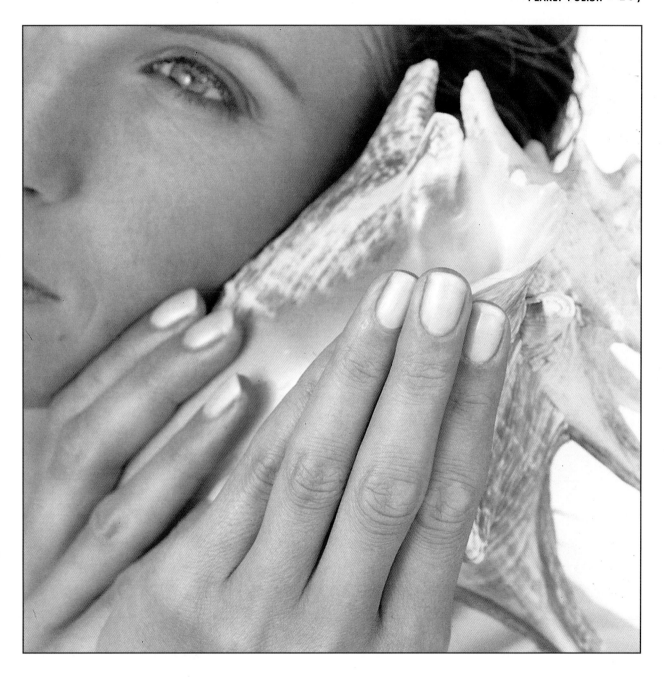

Bright and Beautiful

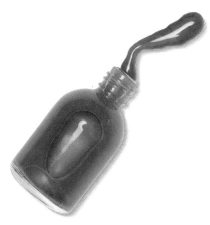

Above: These days, coloured polishes break all the rules.

Below: Try painting a different colour on to each nail.

Nail polish colours have gone through a revolution recently. Now you're not just confined to reds and pinks. These days, you can buy a kaleidoscope of wild and wacky shades – from green to yellow, blue to silver. The choice is yours.

MAKING THE MOST OF BRIGHT COLOURS

■ Bright nail polish stains nails, so first apply at least one coat of clear base coat to prevent this from happening.

■ For fun, paint a different colour on to each nail – or alternate two colours.

■ Keep the rest of your make-up simple, or you'll end up with a really overpowering look!

■ If you're going to draw attention to your nails by using bright colours, they have to be in great condition. Indulge them with a weekly manicure.

■ Metallic finishes are very popular, but can be quite drying on the nails. Use a nourishing base coat underneath to prevent this, and go bare-nailed at least one day a week. If you do end up with stains on your nails, scrub them with a little facial scrub, then lightly buff the surface.

■ Even though they look dramatic in the bottle, some polishes look disappointingly sheer on the nail. You'll need to apply a few coats to build up the effect.

Right: Even if the rest of your make-up is subtle, your nails can be in striking colours.

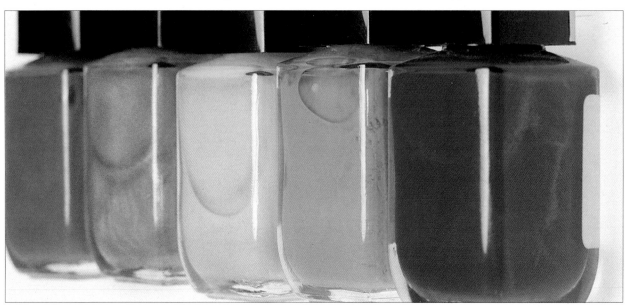

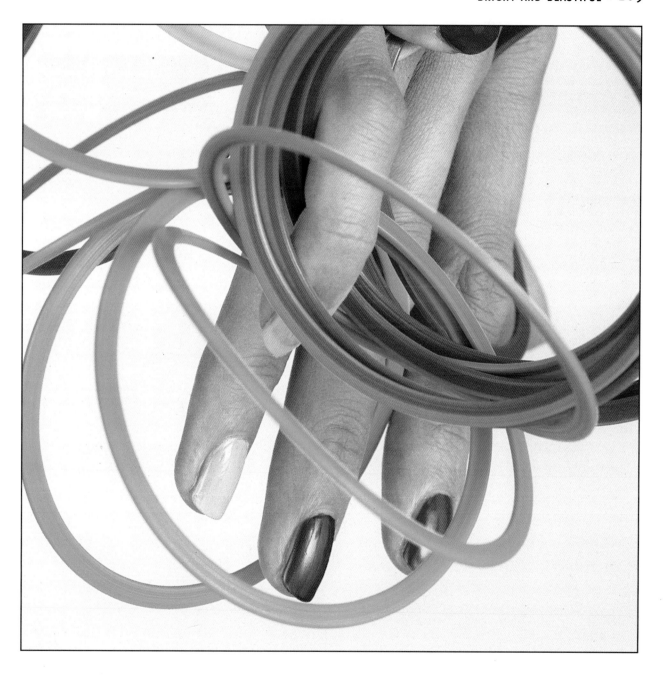

Get the Glitter Bug!

Once you've mastered some basic manicure techniques, have some fun and try some glittery looks.

■ Look out in stationery shops for larger glitter shapes, such as the stars used here (see far right). Pick up a single star shape with a pair of eyebrow tweezers and drop in place on a wet nail. Use the tip of the tweezer to ensure that it's secured. Again, apply a coat of clear polish to hold it in place for longer.

■ Some nail polishes have glitter already blended into them. The more coats you apply, the more glittery the finish will be.

■ A great way to add instant sparkle to ordinary nail polish is by sprinkling on a little loose glitter. Just sprinkle it over wet nail polish and leave to dry. Paint a clear coat of polish over the top to hold it in place for longer.

■ Another way to give your nails a pretty, speckled look is to apply a coat of bold colour and allow it to dry. Use a toothpick to dot a contrasting colour on the top.

Below: Liven up a clear polish with a sprinkling of glitter.

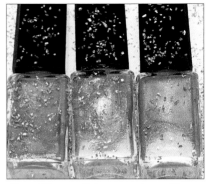

Above: These polishes come in a wide range of colours.

Right: Star spangled nails steal the show!

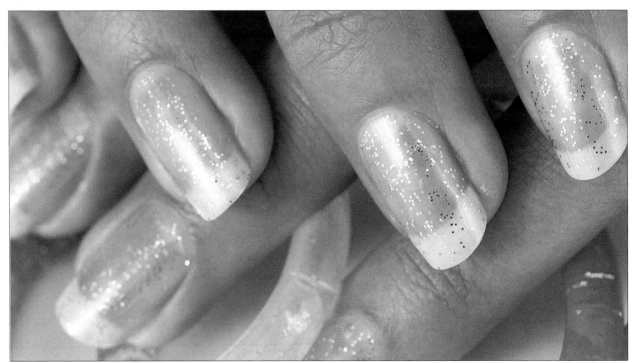

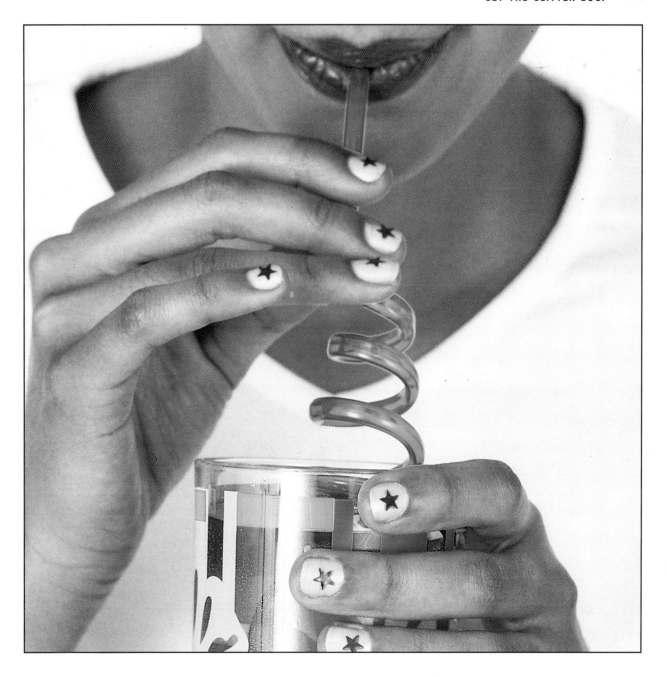

Fake It!

Artificial nails were first developed in Hollywood in the 1930s using basic plastics which were fine for photographic purposes but looked false in real life. Today's false nails are much more sophisticated, tougher and less likely to damage the nail underneath. There are four main types of false nails to choose from, depending on whether you want to replace a broken nail or have the instant gratification of a complete set of false nails.

Stick-on nails

These are precast plastic nail shapes that you apply with a special fixative or double-sided tape. They can be applied at home and look natural so long as you choose the right size. Most suppliers offer stick-on nails in a variety of nail widths.

Brush-on acrylic nails

The surface of the nail is first roughened and then the acrylic chemical is painted on and allowed to dry. It can then be styled into the desired shape. It grows out with your own nail. It is best carried out by a professional manicurist.

Nail extensions

These are made of plastic and are bonded to your nails with a special glue to ensure that they stay in place until your nail grows out. They can be filed as your nails get longer. Again, these are best applied by a professional manicurist.

Nail wrapping

This technique is used to reattach a broken nail tip to the nail or extend the length of your nails. A combination of fine tissue papers and fast drying glue is used to build up your nails. This is best left to a professional manicurist for good results.

Right: False nails can look as good as the real thing.

Below left: Take care to match the false stick-on nail to the shape of the nail bed.

Below: Nail wrapping is a technique which combines fine tissue papers and fast drying glue to build up your nails.

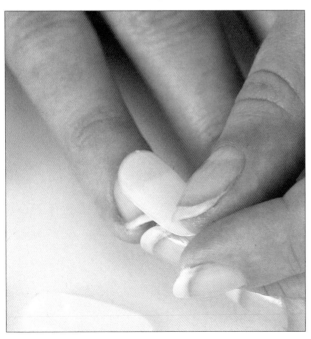

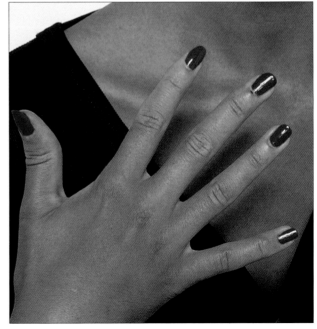

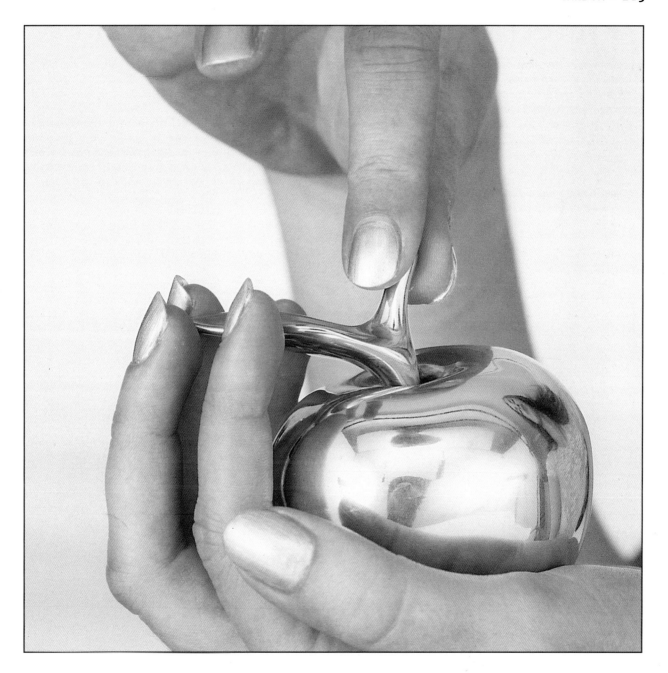

Protective Care for Summer Hands

Your hands need some extra special care when temperatures rise. The good news is, just a little special attention will ensure that they look their best at home or abroad.

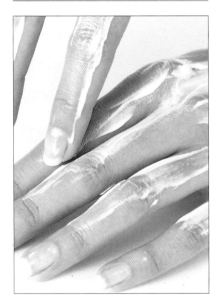

Above: Regular moisturizing with a sunscreen lotion or hand cream keeps the ageing effects of the sun at bay. Use all year round for maximum protection from the sun's ultraviolet rays.

THE SUNNY SIDE OF HANDCARE

■ Exposure to the sun is the main cause of skin ageing. In fact, experts believe that it's responsible for up to 90% of the visible signs of aging. Even if you're in your teens, it's essential to protect your hands from the ageing effects of the sun, because the damage you do now won't be evident for many years. Whatever your age, smooth the backs of your hands with a sunscreen lotion or a hand cream that filters out the sun's harmful ultraviolet rays. This will also help guard against the dangers of skin cancer – commonly found on the backs of hands because they face so much daily exposure.

■ Every night, apply a dot of nail strengthener oil to your nails, then apply your usual hand cream.

■ When you apply suntan lotion, rub a little into your nails. The oils will help counteract the drying effects of the sun.

■ Before starting to do gardening, first scrape your nails over a bar of soap or soapy nail brush. The undersides of your nails will fill up with soap, acting as a barrier against dirt, grime and infection.

■ Holidays are the perfect time to experiment with new polish colours. Tropical colours and pearly whites look great against lightly tanned fingers.

Right: Hot weather tactics make for beautiful nails.

Below: Try scraping your nails over soap or a soapy nail brush before gardening.

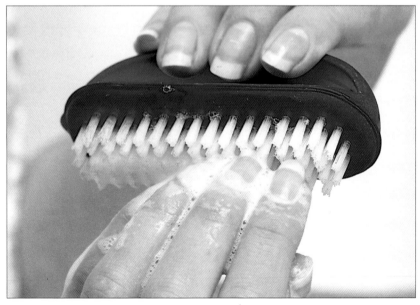

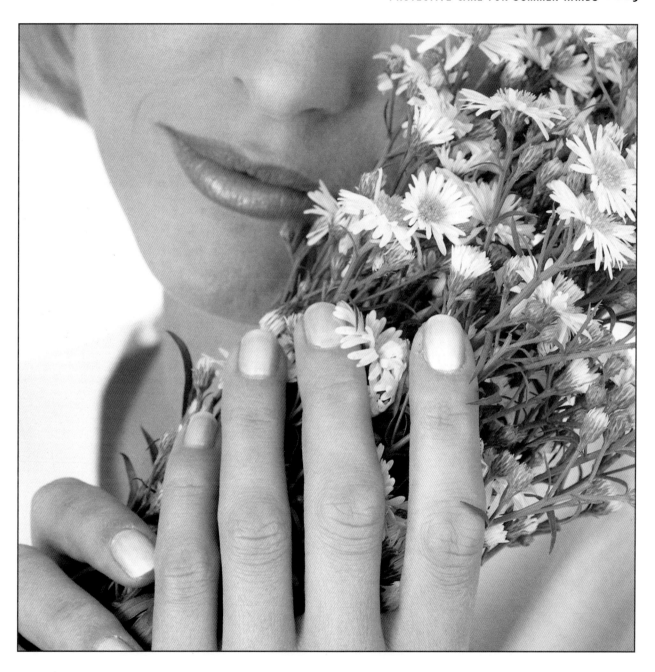

Soothing Care for Winter Hands

Freezing temperatures, biting winds and central heating can literally strip the skin on your hands of their natural oils. It can also weaken your nails, leaving them dry and flaky. Just as you need to lavish extra care on your face and body at this time of year, the same applies to your hands.

ICE MAIDEN TACTICS

The low concentration of oil glands in the back of your hands means that this area lacks natural protection. In winter, frequent washing and contact with detergents makes them even more vulnerable than your face. Choose a hand cream that contains a high level of protection and apply by massaging it into your hands first, then working up to your wrists. Just as your skin needs a richer moisturizer at this time of year, your hands may also need a more nourishing hand cream, so switch from runny liquids to thick creams. Thicker creams also have a higher oil content that will help seal extra moisture into the upper layers of your skin.

■ Take extra care to dry your hands thoroughly after washing. Any remaining dampness on the skin will freeze in the cold air, leading to soreness and chapping.

■ Treat your hands to a hand mask. You can either use a moisturizing face mask or improvise with a rich hand cream. Simply smooth over your hands, working the cream right down to the tips of your nails. Leave to soak into your skin for 10-20 minutes. Then wipe off the excess and rub in any residue.

■ Protect your hands from the outside elements by investing in warm gloves.

■ If you have weak nails, use a cotton-bud (swab) with a pointed end to clean under the free edge – it's gentler than scrubbing with a nail brush.

Right: Beautiful hands – even when temperatures fall below zero.

Below left: Lavish your hands with the same care as you give your complexion and you will soon reap the benefits!

Below: Switch to a richer cream to increase your skin's moisture levels.

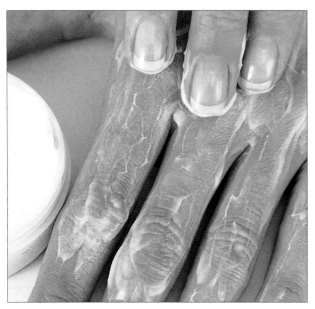

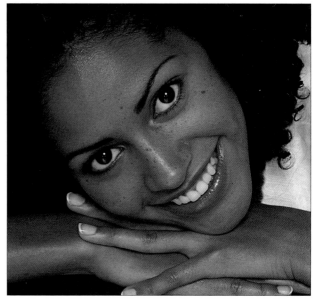

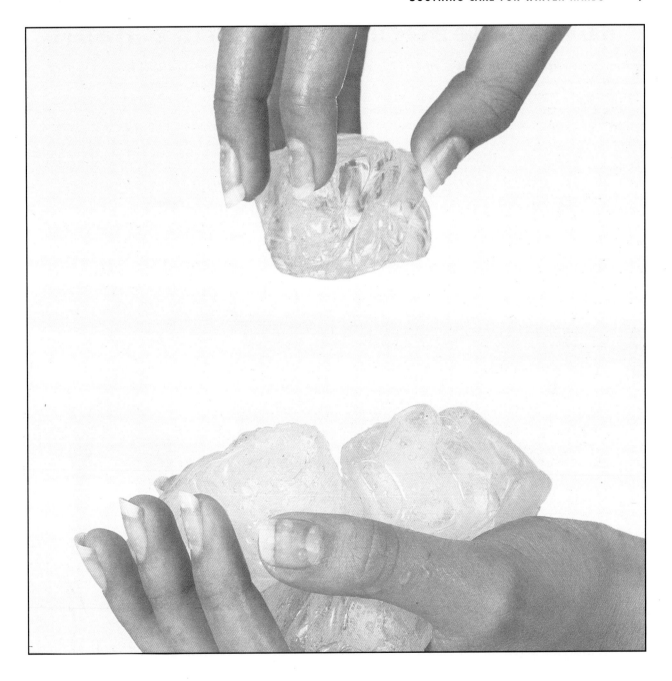

How to Beat the Nail Biting Habit

The most expensive manicure in the world will be worthless if you bite your nails. It's a very hard habit to break, but one worth beating if you're serious about having beautiful hands and nails.

TIPS TO STOP NAIL BITING

■ Devote 10 minutes a day to caring for your nails. As your nails look a bit better, you'll be more inclined to stick with it.

■ Try one of the anti-bite lotions that are on the market. Once you've stopped for a couple of weeks, your longer nails will give you the incentive to keep up the good work.

■ If you have short nails, it doesn't mean you shouldn't use nail polish. Even the stubbiest, shortest nails look better for an application of clear or pale pearly polish.

■ Consider wearing false nails for a while so your nails have a chance to grow underneath. Even the most determined of nail biters have trouble gnawing through them! Just a few weeks is often all it takes to break the habit.

■ Some former nail biters say that restricting themselves to just one nail can do the trick. Once you see how nice the other nails look, you'll be inspired to grow out the bitten one.

■ If you bite your nails because you're feeling stressed or nervous, try playing with a set of worry beads instead.

■ Use scented hand cream – the taste of the perfume will put you off biting!

> **Tip**
> Carry a nail file with you at all times. That way you can instantly smooth away straggly edges that will tempt you to bite.

Right: Break the biting habit for beautiful nails.

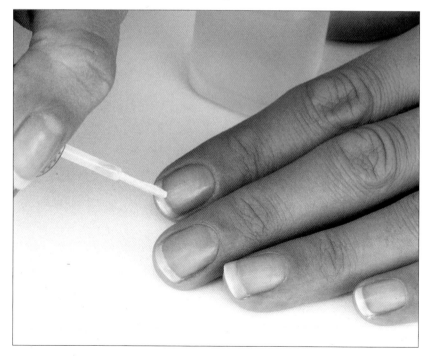

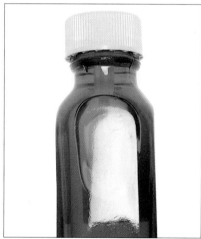

Above: Invest in an anti-bite lotion. Just one nibble could put you off the biting habit for life!

Left: Apply the anti-bite lotion every day to ensure success.

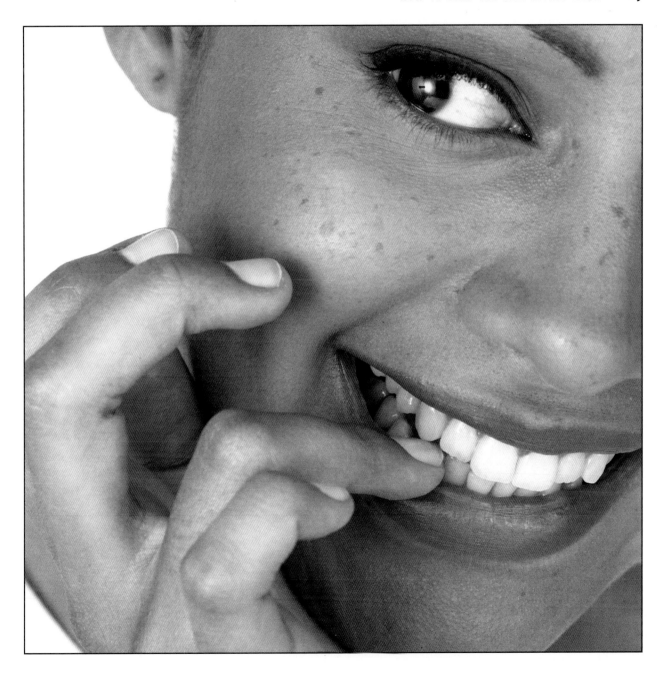

20 Quick Tips for Beautiful Hands

It's often the small things that make all the difference to the way your nails look.

1 Pay for your manicure beforehand – rummaging for cash can ruin fresh polish.

2 Dunk freshly polished nails into a bowl of iced water to help polish dry quickly.

3 To extend the life of your polish, clean the top of the bottle with a tissue after applying – polish buildup allows air into the bottle and the product evaporates.

4 Cheap nail polishes thicken with age – dilute them with a base coat to make them last longer.

5 Prolong the life of your manicure by painting on a top coat every other day.

6 Make a polish last longer by washing your nails in warm soapy water. Then wipe your nails thoroughly with a tissue to remove any residues before applying a layer of polish.

7 Ink or nicotine stains can be bleached away by rubbing your fingers with a slice of neat lemon. Rub in lots of hand cream afterwards to counteract the drying effects.

8 Dry nails quickly by blasting gently with the cool air flow button of your hair dryer.

9 Store nail polishes in the refrigerator to prevent them from becoming too thick – it helps prevent evaporation and the polish stays liquid for longer.

10 Rub a little petroleum jelly around the neck of a new bottle of polish to prevent it from sticking in future.

11 When removing nail polish, swish the cotton wool (cotton balls) from the base of your nail to the tip so you don't have to push drying nail polish remover into your delicate cuticles.

12 Don't just use the tip of the brush when applying polish or you'll risk applying too much polish. The brush should be splayed out against the nail horizontally. This means you'll get thinner, more even layers of polish – which means a more professional finish.

13 Don't apply polish in the sunshine – the polish will bubble as it dries.

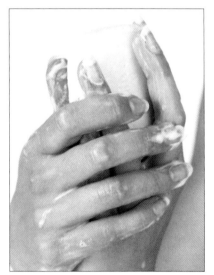

Above: Lather up before a manicure to ensure streak-free nails.

Right: A base coat over and under the nail will help to strengthen it.

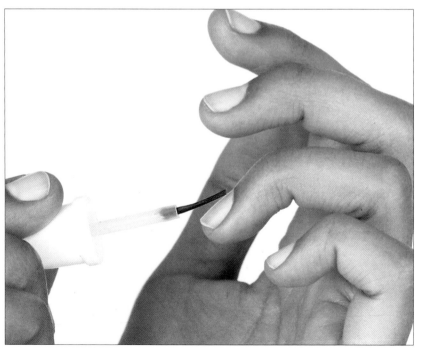

14 If you mess up a nail and you're pressed for time, you don't have to take off all the polish. Instead, dampen the pad of your opposite index finger with nail polish remover and pat over the messy nail. The globby polish will smooth out sufficiently so you can let it dry and apply polish over it.

15 Apply a mud face pack to the backs of your hands for deep-down cleansing. Apply lots of nourishing hand cream afterwards.

16 Remove any traces of polish on surrounding skin with a cottonbud (swab) dipped in nail polish remover.

17 For the illusion of longer, slimmer nails, leave a very slight space at either side of the nail when painting.

18 If you've run out of polish remover, try this tip: coat your nail with some clear base coat. Let it set for 45 seconds, then press cotton wool (cotton balls) over the nail and remove – the base coat and colour will come off in one fell swoop.

19 Paint your base coat up and around the tip of the nail to strengthen your nails and help prevent breakages.

20 A pumice stone is not just for feet! Using one gently on your hands is a good way to remove ingrained dirt and stains.

Below left: Sweep off polish from base to tip to protect your cuticles.

Below: A top coat will keep nails looking good every day.

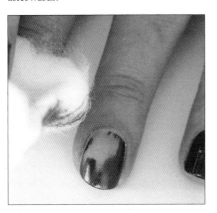

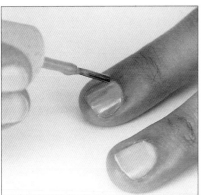

Above: Apply polish thinly. Several thin coats of polish give a more professional finish than one or two thick layers.

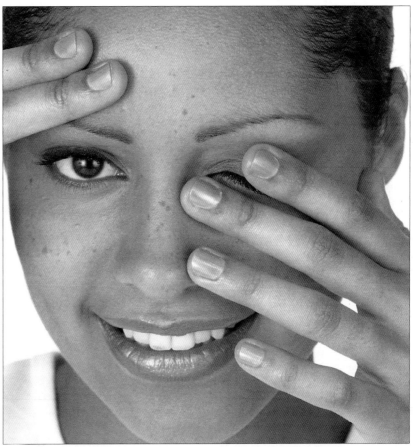

Manicure Q&A

Whatever your nailcare problems, we've got the answers!

Q: "The tips of my nails look discoloured. What can I do about them?"
A: Dip a cottonbud (swab) in some neat lemon juice and work it under the nail. Leave for 10 minutes. Rinse well afterwards and apply lots of hand cream to counteract the drying effects.

Q: "I've noticed that some nail polishes are labelled as hypo-allergenic and suitable for sensitive skins. Surely your nails can't be allergic to nail polish?"
A: Your nails aren't but your skin can be! Remember that we constantly touch our faces with our hands throughout the day. If you're sensitive to the ingredients in nail polish, you may set up a reaction – such as red, inflamed skin around your eyes, lips and nose. However, hypo-allergenic nail polish is less likely to set off an irritation because the ingredients that are likely to cause it have been removed.

Q: "Costume jewellery causes an allergic reaction on my fingers. Is there anything I can do, without having to throw it out?"
A: Coat the inside of the jewellery with some hypo-allergenic clear nail polish. Also, make sure you're not building up a residue of soap under your rings, which can irritate the skin.

Q: "Is there anything I can do to get rid of ridges on my nails?"
A: Most nails have ridges in the surface, running from the cuticle to the tip. If they're quite prominent, you can gently buff the surface of your nail with a nail buffer to make them less obvious. However, go gently and take care not to

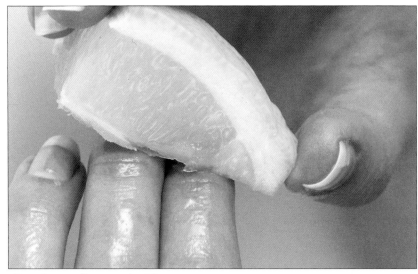

Above: Say goodbye to stained fingers with a slice of lemon. Rub the lemon juice and rind over the stained area.

thin the nails. Most nailcare companies also offer a product called a ridge filler, which you apply under your nail polish to fill in the ridges and create a smoother surface on which to work.

Q: "Why does a nail turn black if it's been damaged?"
A: If you trap your finger in a door, it will turn black because the nail bed bleeds. The blood has nowhere to go, so dries and attaches itself to the nail bed. You can lessen the effects by dunking your damaged finger in ice cold water to help stop the bleeding.

Q: "Is there anything I can do to get rid of nicotine or ink stains on my fingers?"
A: Rub half a lemon (both juice and rind) over the affected area. If stains are persistent, try lightly buffing with a nail buffer.

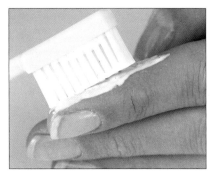

Above: Applying toothpaste with a brush helps to remove nicotine or ink stains.

Alternatively, try applying a touch of toothpaste with a brush.

Right: The French manicure looks good with everything.

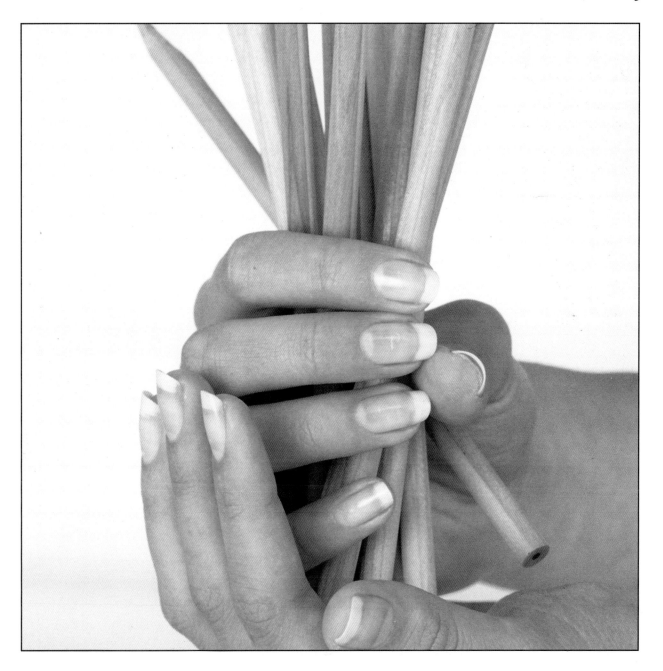

Foot Notes

Anyone can have pretty feet if they give them some attention. But the truth of the matter is, most of us ignore our feet until we want to wear revealing shoes or open-toe sandals. However, feet respond best to a little care every day rather than a major blitz every once in a while. So, kick off your shoes and give your feet the pampering they deserve!

PLAYING FOOTSIE

This is the essential kit you need to ensure that your feet get the TLC they deserve:

Nail clippers
Using nail clippers is the best way to cut the thick nails on your feet without causing any splitting.

Emery board
This is used to smooth away any hard edges after clipping your toenails. Look for longer ones, as it'll be easier to reach your toes.

Toe separators
These allow you to apply polish to your nails without smudging it on to your toes.

Pumice stone
This is used to gently rub away patches of hard skin from the soles and sides of your feet.

Foot lotion
Apply this every day to keep the skin on your feet soft and smooth, and to help avoid a buildup of hard skin.

Cuticle cream
Rub over the cuticles of your toenails once a week to soften them and make them easier to push back.

Hoof stick
The rubber tip of a hoof stick helps you to gently push cuticles back after applying cuticle cream.

Clear polish
Just one coat of clear, shiny colour on your toenails will make your feet look better.

Polish remover
Use to remove old polish before applying a new coat.

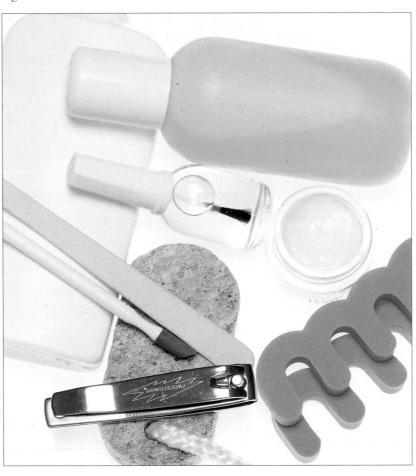

DID YOU KNOW?

■ There are 26 bones and 115 ligaments in each foot, as well as tendons and muscles, all of which are arranged to create several dynamic arches that support the body weight.

■ On average, we take 18,000 steps a day.

■ Each time our feet hit the floor, double the weight of our body impacts with the floor.

■ Over 50% of women don't like their feet, probably as a result of foot problems. The good news is that you can do things to make your feet look more attractive.

■ Our feet contain around 250,000 sweat glands and they perspire more than any other part of our body. On average, each foot produces an eggcupful (a 1/2 cup) of sweat each day.

■ In our lifetime, it's estimated that our feet carry us an average of 70,000 miles (112,000 km) — or almost three times around the world.

■ The average foot size has increased over the past 100 years from size 3 (5 USA) to size 6 (8 USA).

Left: Everything you need for pretty feet. Clockwise from bottom left: pumice stone; clippers; hoof stick; emery board; foot lotion; polish remover; clear polish; cuticle cream; toe separators.

Right: Feet respond best to a little care every day — regular care makes feet fit to flaunt.

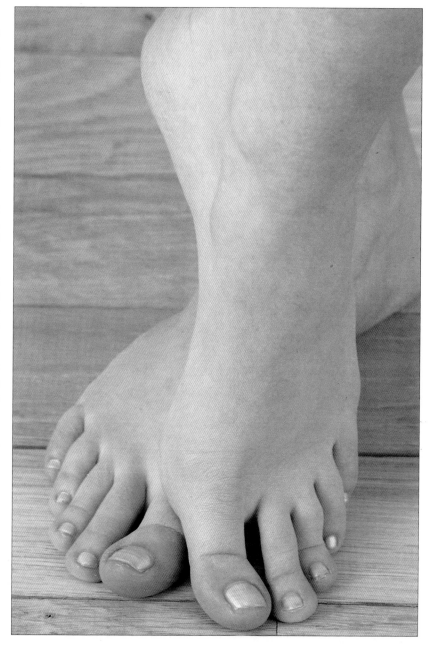

Easy Steps to Softer Feet

Considering the punishment they take, it's no wonder that feet develop areas of hard skin and callouses. These tips will help keep the skin soft, supple and smooth.

■ Soak your feet in a bowl of warm soapy water to soften hard skin.

■ To really soften areas of rough skin, add 30ml/2 tbsp of bicarbonate of soda (baking soda) to the warm water. Soak your feet for 15 minutes before setting to work with a pumice stone.

■ Smooth away problem areas with a foot file or pumice stone. Work over the heels, sides and soles of your feet, but leave the toes well alone.

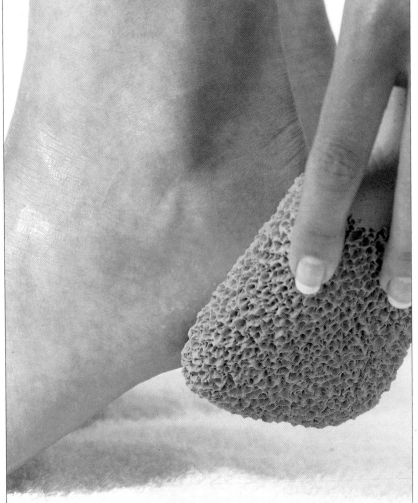

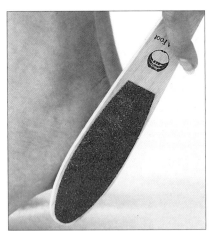

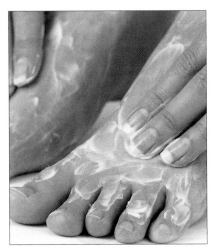

■ If you don't have a pumice stone, use an ordinary body scrub instead.

■ The secret of dealing with hard skin is to gently rub it away every day rather than trying to remove it in one session. Otherwise, you'll risk ending up with red, sore feet.

■ Apply foot cream to your feet every day, rubbing it in well and avoiding the spaces between the toes. Take the time to knead and massage every inch of the sole, heel and top side of the foot.

■ If you have a big buildup of hard skin, you should see a qualified chiropodist rather than trying to remove it yourself.

■ Once a week, rub your feet with a thick layer of cream, pull on a pair of socks and head for bed. Your feet will be much softer in the morning.

Far left: Use a pumice stone, a foot scrub or a foot file to remove any hard skin and keep your feet healthy. Concentrate on the parts of your feet where hard skin builds up – especially the heels.

Top left: A foot file is another alternative to a pumice stone.

Left: Treat your feet to a regular relaxing massage.

Right: A foot bath provides a soothing heat – and an effective cure for hard skin, too.

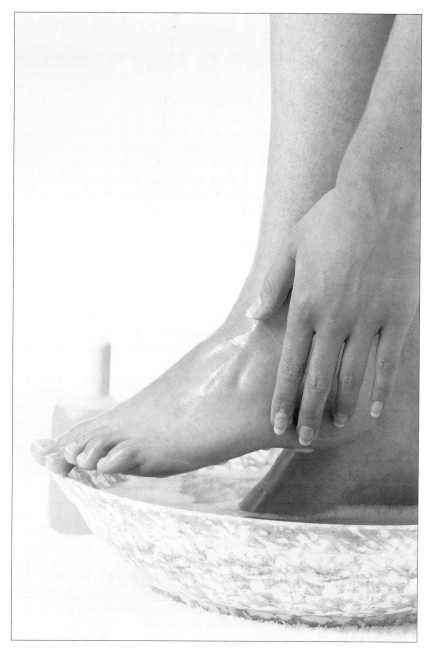

The Quick and Easy Pedicure

This weekly pedicure will ensure that your toenails always look presentable.

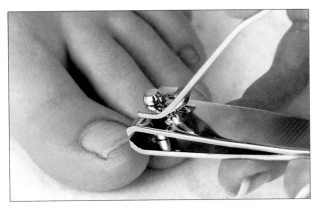

1 Cut off any excess toenail with a pair of nail clippers, working straight across the nail. Avoid using nail scissors as these can split the nail and cause ingrowing toenails.

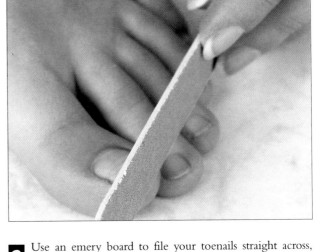

2 Use an emery board to file your toenails straight across, rounding them slightly at the corners. To avoid ingrowing toenails, don't file into the corners of the nails. Hold the board slightly angled down towards the free edge of the nail and smooth from each side of the nail towards the centre.

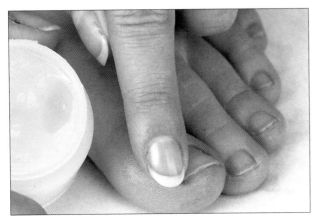

3 Massage a little cuticle cream into the base of your nails.

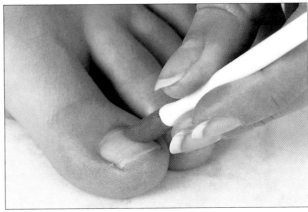

4 Push back your cuticle with a hoof stick or a cottonbud (swab). Use circular movements for greatest effect. Wipe off any excess cream, and finish with a coat of clear nail polish.

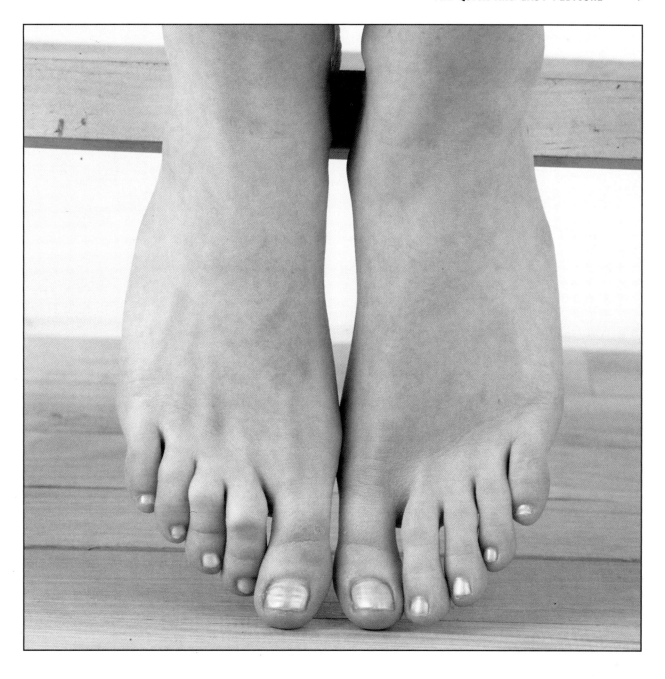

Fancy Footwork

If you love bright-coloured nail polishes but find they're too overpowering on your fingernails, then try wearing them on your toes! A flash of bright colour under sandals or mules will instantly brighten up a summer or evening look.

TIPS FOR PAINTED TOENAILS

■ If your feet and toes aren't your best feature, it's a good idea to try a clear, pearlized or pale-coloured nail polish so you don't draw too much attention to them.

■ Because your feet have to be pushed into shoes, polish often gets smudged on your toenails. Even if the polish is dry to the touch, it's still liable to be wet for a few hours after application. It's best to paint your toenails when you know you won't need to wear shoes for a while.

Right: Sponge toe separators stop your polish smudging.

Far right: If your feet look good, show them off with bright polish.

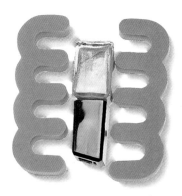

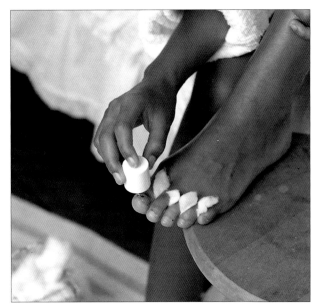

Above: Before you apply nail polish, try separating your toes either with a foam rubber separator, by using cotton wool (cotton balls), or twist a tissue into a narrow strip and weave it in and out of your toes to prevent smudging. Apply a clear base coat to create a smooth surface on which to work and to prevent bright nail polishes from staining your toenails. Then apply two coats of coloured nail polish.

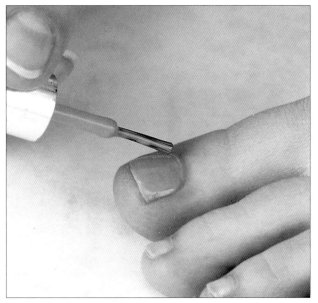

Above: Work each nail by painting a stripe of colour down the centre, and then overlapping with a strip of colour down each side. Leave each coat to dry thoroughly. Apply a clear top coat to seal in the colour and make it extra hardwearing. Leave it to dry as long as you can before putting on your shoes. At least an hour is recommended as even socks and tights can leave their imprints if put on too soon.

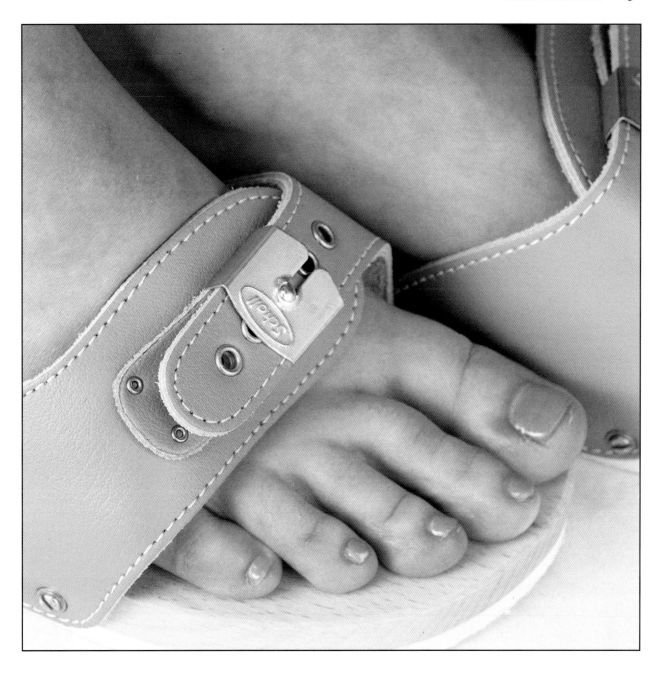

Pedicure Q&A

We've got the answers to your foot-care problems!

Q: "How can I be sure I'm choosing the right size shoes?"
A: Try these tips:
■ Feel your foot through the leather to ensure a comfortable fit. Bulges can be a sign that there is pressure on a toe.

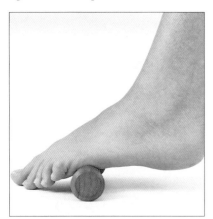

Above: Try rolling your feet over a foot massager after a long, hard day.

■ Take a short walk wearing the shoe and check for slipping or gaping.
■ Never buy shoes you know are too small in the hope they'll stretch – they'll definitely damage your feet.
■ Buy shoes in the late afternoon when your feet are at their largest.
■ If your feet tend to swell in summer, try sandals on when your feet are swollen or buy half a size larger.
■ Shoes should have good support under the heel and instep and have enough room for the feet to spread inside the shoes.

■ High heels throw the body's alignment off balance, so wear them as little as possible. Choose shoes with a low heel and a flexible sole to allow the ligaments and muscles of the sole to be exercised.
Q: "Is there anything I can do to perk my feet up at the end of a hard day?"
A: Any of these tips will help:
■ Lie down with your feet higher than your head for 10 minutes.
■ Roll your feet over a foot massager. It will improve the circulation in your feet.
■ Massage your feet with a tingling mint foot gel.
■ Give your feet a friction rub with a towel, then massage them with cologne – it'll feel wonderful as it evaporates.
■ Sit on the edge of the bath with your feet under the tap at full pressure. Start with warm water, increase to hot, then gradually turn to cold. Stay there for as long as you can, then dry your feet.

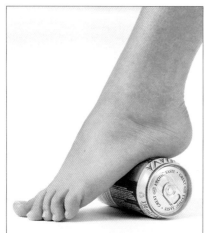

Above: Roll your feet over a can of cold drink straight from the refrigerator!

Q: "How can I make sure my trainers (sneakers) give my feet the protection they need?"
A: Check that they fulfil these conditions:
■ They should be lightweight with adequate cushioning to absorb impact on landing and reduce stress on the joints.
■ They should support your feet to help prevent twists and strains. The kind of shoe you choose depends on the exercise you're doing. For instance, aerobics shoes have extra support in the arches and on the outside. It's worth buying a pair of cross trainers (sneakers) if you do several different types of activities. Whatever you do, buy your shoes at a good sports store where the staff can advise you on the best shoe for your needs.
■ Take your last pair of trainers (sneakers) with you, so the shop assistant can see which part of the shoe you wear down the most and then advise you properly.

Right: Perfect care for pretty feet.

Below: Spritz your feet with a deodorizing foot spray before putting on your shoes in the morning.

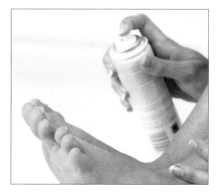

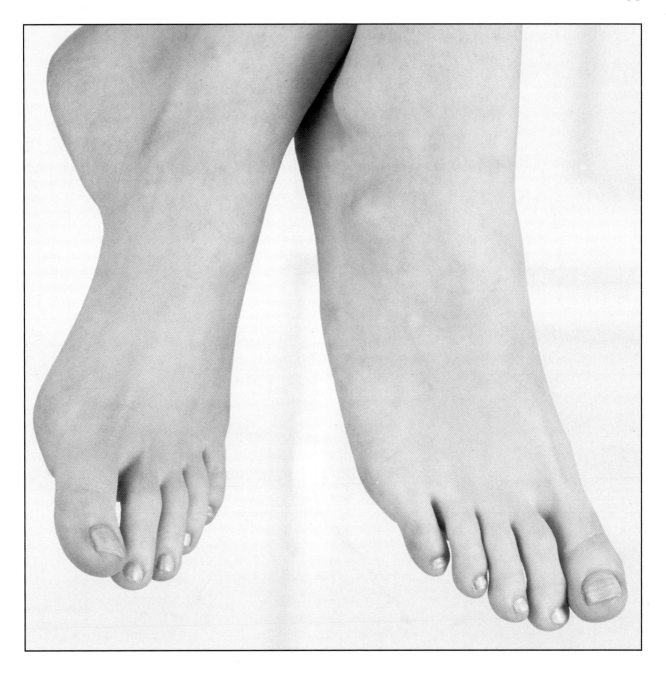

Manicure and Pedicure Buzzwords

This is a brief A to Z of manicure and pedicure words. If you're not sure what it means, look it up here:

Athlete's foot

A highly contagious fungal infection that thrives in damp warm areas of the skin, especially between the toes. The skin splits and is accompanied by an itchy rash. There are good treatments that you can buy at the chemist, but consult your doctor if the condition doesn't clear up. To avoid it in the first place, wear flip flops in communal changing rooms, don't share towels and keep feet clean and dry between washes.

Bunion

An enlargement of the toe joint, usually on the big toe. It's usually caused by shoes that are too tight and is often very painful.

Calluses

General patches of hard skin on the feet caused by an uneven displacement of

Below: Use a pumice stone every day.

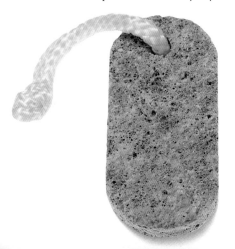

body weight. Guard against them by wearing comfortable shoes and using a pumice stone to rub away dry spots of skin as they appear.

Corns

Usually found on the toes, corns develop as a result of pressure or friction. You can buy corn pads at the chemist; but see a qualified chiropodist if they don't clear up.

Cuticle

The thin strip of skin that protects the living cells under your nail from any possible infection.

Hangnails

Pieces of skin torn away from but still attached to the base or side of a fingernail. They're usually caused when the cuticles have dried and cracked.

Hoof stick

A manicure stick with a rubber tip used to push back your cuticles.

Ingrowing toenail

Incorrect trimming and filing of the nails can cause the edge to grow into the skin. These are usually very painful and should be treated by a doctor or chiropodist. Don't be tempted to ease or cut the nail yourself or you'll risk infection.

Keratin

A protein substance that forms the base of your nails.

Lunula

Also known as the "half moon" at the base of your nails.

Leuconychia

These white spots are either caused by general wear and tear or by blows to the matrix of the nail. They grow out naturally with the nail.

Matrix

The area just beneath the cuticle where new nail cells are formed. It's the actively growing tissue.

Nail plate

The visible part of the nail that rests on the nail bed.

Verruca

A highly contagious viral wart-like infection found on the sole of the foot. The surface of the skin appears rough or granular, often with small black dots in the centre. You can usually get rid of them by using remedies from the chemist. If they persist, have them checked or removed by your doctor.

Right: Hands and feet to be proud of.

Below: Scrub up your act.

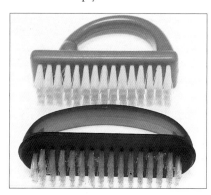

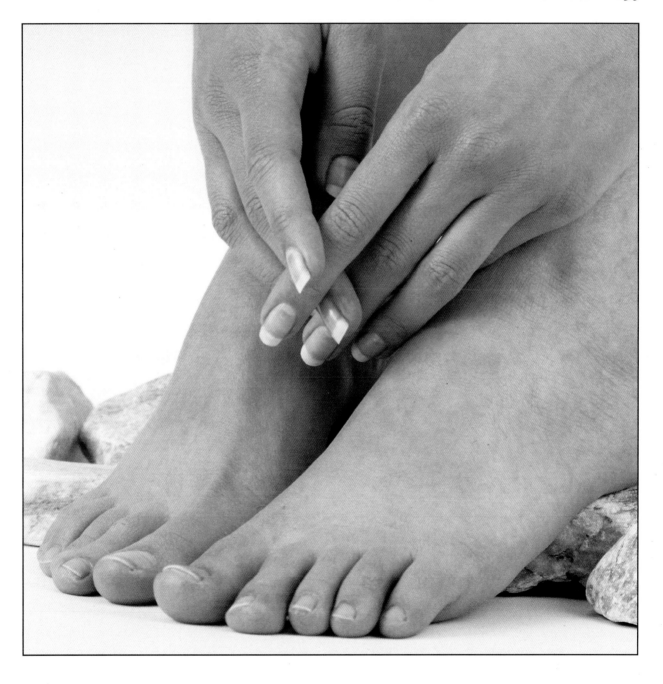

Diet and Exercise

A well-balanced diet is the secret to being in good
health and great shape. But eating well does not mean
you have to buy expensive foods or cook time-
consuming meals. If your current diet includes too
many "wrong" foods, be practical about revamping it,
and don't be too tough on yourself – it is not a crime
to enjoy forbidden foods from time to time. The same
goes for diet and exercise. Get into the habit of eating
a low fat diet and combine it with regular exercise,
and you will have no problems getting into shape.

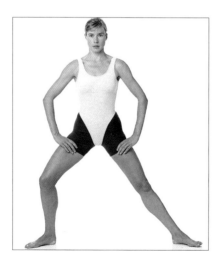

Above: Take up regular exercise and get
the fitness bug!

Right: Eating fresh fruit on a daily basis
will benefit you from head to toe.

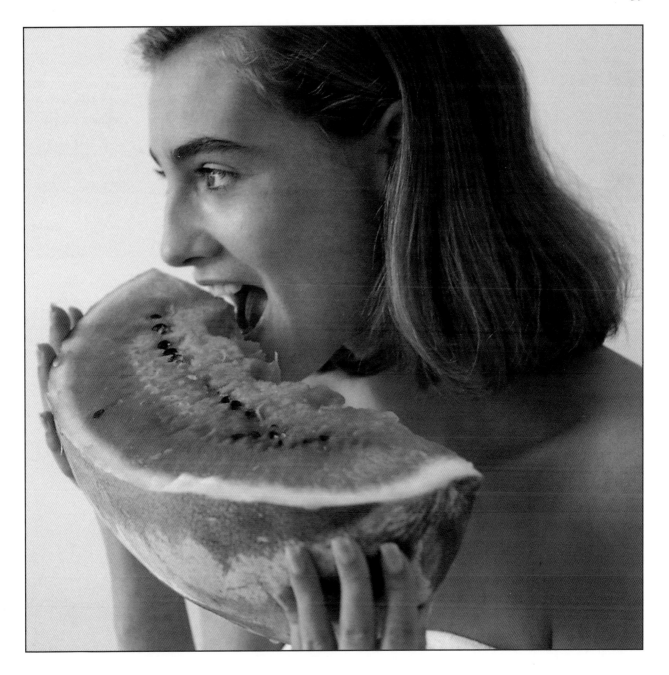

Diet for Life

Balance is important to a healthy diet. The way we eat affects our well-being, so knowing how to choose a healthy combination of foods is the first step towards improving our eating habits and lifestyle.

FAT – FRIEND AND FOE

Eggs, butter, milk, and meat are a good source of fat, but we tend to eat too much of it which is why many of us are overweight: fat produces fat. Cut down on fat in your diet but do not cut it out completely: eat less fatty red meat and more fish and poultry; grill, bake, or stir-fry (using polyunsaturated and monounsaturated oils), eat eggs in moderation, and use semi-skimmed or skimmed milk instead of full-fat milk. Try to use margarine, or try switching to a reduced fat olive-oil spread instead of butter; if you really can't live without butter, reserve it for special occasions.

Saturated fats come mainly from animal products (milk, butter, cheese, and meat) and, in excess, are thought to contribute to raised cholesterol levels.

Polyunsaturated fats are found in vegetable oils such as sunflower, corn, safflower, and soya bean oils; they are also found in some fish oils and some nuts. Polyunsaturated fats are said to help lower cholesterol levels.

Monounsaturated fats are found in olive and rapeseed oils; they are also said to lower cholesterol levels.

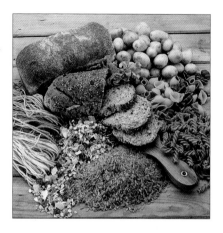

Above: Get healthy with cereals and grains.

GRAINS, FRUIT, AND VEGETABLES

Eat plenty of wholemeal (whole-wheat) foods such as brown rice, wholemeal bread, wholemeal flour, and wholemeal pasta; they should form the bulk of a healthy diet. Concentrate on eating lots of fresh fruit and vegetables.

SUGAR SWEET

Many of us eat too much sugar, so try cutting added sugar out of your diet completely for 21 days (your body will still obtain it naturally from certain vegetables and fruit) and see how you feel: even if you are not actively dieting you will probably find that you lose some weight. Some women find that they crave sugary foods when pre-menstrual. One way of combating this is to eat little and often; snack on fruit with a high water content, such as watermelon and strawberries.

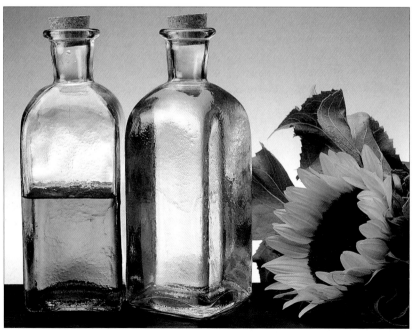

Left: Choose vegetable oils for cooking.

SALTY ISSUES

Even if you are not dieting you should eat less salt as it may lead to high blood pressure. Good low-sodium salts are available, so use these instead of the real thing to season food. Do not buy salted butter, avoid processed and smoked cheeses and processed foods, and add the barest minimum of salt to cooking water.

FLUID INTAKE

Drink plenty of water: your body loses between 2–3 litres/3–5 pints of fluid every day, so drink no less than 1.5 litres/ 2½ pints of water daily. Once you get into the swing of it, consciously drinking water is easy – just keep some to hand and sip it slowly throughout the day.

HEALTHY DIET CHECKLIST

The guidelines shown here are not difficult to apply, and they will soon become part of your daily routine.

■ Eat lots of fresh fruit and vegetables.

■ Be wary of the amount of fat you eat.

■ Eat half your daily food in the form of starchy carbohydrates such as potatoes, bread, pasta and rice.

■ Eat fibre-rich foods such as wholemeal (whole-wheat) bread, pasta and pulses.

■ Cut down on sugar and salt.

■ Drink more water and swap coffee and tea for herbal teas.

■ Cut down on sugary drinks and alcohol intake. Limit yourself to 14 units a week, the same as 2 glasses of wine a day.

IDEAL WEEKLY FOOD QUOTA

Try to eat foods from each of the four main food groups each day.

■ Starchy carbohydrate foods, including bread, cereals, pasta, potatoes and rice.

■ Dairy products (preferably low fat).

■ Protein foods – meat, fish, poultry, beans and lentils, nuts and eggs.

■ Vegetables and fruit. Eating 5 portions a day from this group is thought to help prevent cancer.

EATING FOR ENERGY

Do you often feel tired and lethargic? Does your energy dip dramatically in the afternoons, making you feel sleepy? If this sounds like you and you want to take action, one of the wisest things to do is to look at your diet and, if necessary, change what you eat and how you eat it.

OFF TO A GOOD START

There is much logic behind the saying "breakfast like a king, lunch like a prince and dine like a pauper". If you start the day with a substantial breakfast your body will get all the energy it needs early on.

CHANGING YOUR EATING HABITS

You will be more successful in changing your diet if you eat regularly, in moderation, and slowly. The bonuses of eating in a balanced way do not come instantly, but if you concentrate on eating fresh foods as well as cutting down alcohol and avoiding high-fat, sugar-rich foods such as cakes, pastries, and salty snacks, you will notice a difference in your energy levels within a few weeks.

VITALITY FOODS FOR EXTRA ENERGY

A diet that makes you feel more energetic is based on natural, wholesome foods that are nutritious, rather than fatty and fast foods. If you want to boost your energy levels, stock up on fresh and dried fruits that are high in natural sugars such as pears, kiwi fruit, and apricots, vegetables such as peas, spinach, cabbage, and onions, and oily fish, poultry, and red meats such as game and lean beef. Eat nuts, brown rice, seeds, pulses, wheatgerm, wholegrains, and foods that contain minerals such as magnesium, phosphorus, and zinc, and water-soluble vitamins B and C. Use cold-pressed oils such as olive, sesame, sunflower, hazelnut, and walnut to dress salads; do not skip dairy foods but use milk and natural yogurt (preferably low fat); replace sliced white loaves with bread made from wholemeal (whole-wheat) flour.

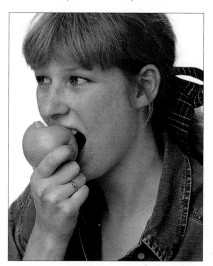

Above: Try to eat fresh fruit every day.

Diet and Weight Loss

People tackle weight loss in ways that suit their lifestyles, but the safest and best way to shift excess pounds is to combine regular exercise with a balanced, calorie-controlled diet. What you eat when you are trying to take off weight should not be that different from a normal eating plan – except for the amount you consume. If you only have a small amount to lose, cut your calorie intake by 1000 from the recommended 2300 calories per day to lose weight. If you are aiming to lose a significant amount, stick to 1200 calories a day and you will get there. Your weight loss ethos should be less sugar and saturated fats, more fibre and starch. The calories you eat should come from foods that supply you with the right number of nutrients to keep your body functioning properly.

MIND OVER MATTER

Quick weight loss is inspiring, but it is important to think ahead too: you need to retrain your palate and eating habits and reassess your physical activity so that you can lose weight and stay slim. You cannot expect to achieve miracles in a few days, but you will see a difference within three or four weeks if you eat properly and exercise regularly. To lose weight successfully you need a horizon – or goal – ahead of you to spur you on.

ABSOLUTELY AVOID

Chocolate, biscuits, doughnuts, fizzy drinks, cakes, sweets, ice cream, sugared cereals – in fact anything that contains refined sugar is just empty calories: a confectionery bar has 230 calories and absolutely no food value.

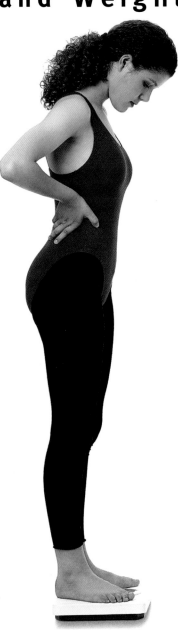

Myth-breaker
If I Stop Smoking Will I Gain Weight?
You may well put on a small amount of weight at first, but if you are serious about getting fitter you have absolutely no choice but to kick smoking. Tobacco is toxic. If you are a smoker, stopping is the biggest leap you can make towards a healthier lifestyle; if you are following a straightforward weight-loss diet and think that kicking the habit will make you pick at food all day, keeps lots of raw vegetables and raisins on hand to munch on.

SLIMMERS' TIPS

■ Eat more at the start of the day to give you energy and time to burn off calories.

■ Eat little and often to stop the hunger pangs. Drinking lots of water also helps.

■ If you need to snack, keep a supply of raw fruit, vegetables, and raisins nearby.

■ Don't take slimming pills, diuretics, or laxatives to speed up weight loss; they upset the body's natural equilibrium and this can take a long time to rebalance.

■ Exercise regularly to use up calories – exercise is essential for weight loss.

■ Don't give up if you lapse: it is quite normal to veer off track every so often. Get back on course as soon as you can, and your hard work will not be ruined.

Left: Don't be tempted to weigh yourself too often – once every 10 days is enough.

Right: Keeping an accurate record of your measurements is one way of calculating weight loss.

HOW MUCH WEIGHT CAN I LOSE?

To lose weight you have to eat fewer calories than your body burns up every day, but the amount varies from person to person. The exact amount depends on how much fat your body has, your metabolism, and the amount you weigh to begin with. As a rule of thumb, the heavier you are when you start slimming, the more weight you are likely to lose within a month. When you lose weight it comes off all areas of your body, but it can take longer to shift from certain areas, such as arms and legs. This is where exercise is helpful: working on specific trouble spots will encourage the weight to come off more quickly.

EATING OUT – AND STAYING ON COURSE

The problem of what to do when dieting and eating out can be a tricky one. The following tips will let you have a good time without lapsing:

■ Order a salad starter and eat the bread roll without the butter.

■ Drink no more than one glass of wine, and, of course, lots and lots of water.

■ Choose a simple main course such as grilled fish or chicken; avoid anything in a rich sauce or in lots of butter.

■ Choose a simple low fat dessert.

■ Finish with herbal tea or espresso or black coffee, not cappuccino.

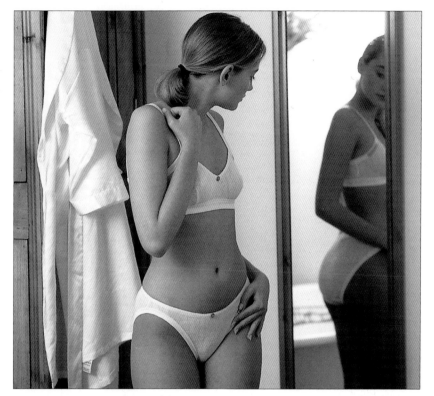

GAUGING WEIGHT LOSS

You may choose to weigh yourself once a week first thing in the morning. Drawing up a goal chart to record any weight losses (and gains) may help to keep you inspired. Or, if you prefer, ignore the scales and just focus on how you feel by keeping a check on how your clothes feel. When tight clothes become more comfortable and noticeably looser, this is a sure sign that you are losing weight. Alternatively, you may prefer to keep a record of your measurements (bust, waist, and hips) and see how they alter over a 28-day period. Do whatever works for you, and when you

have lost a little weight reward yourself with a special calorie-free treat such as a new lipstick, eyeshadow, or a manicure – this is just one positive way to inspire yourself, and to put the pleasure factor back into your life.

> **Myth-breaker**
> **If I Skip Meals Will I Lose Weight More Quickly?**
> Do not be tempted to skip meals. Skipping meals makes you crave, overeat at the next meal, and it slows down your metabolism, which ultimately hinders weight loss.

Body Shape

The shape of your body is unique; it is important to remember this because the basic skeletal and muscular form that you inherit is unchangeable. Features such as your height, foot size, shoulder width and the length and shape of your legs, nose, fingers and toes combine to produce a whole. Each person is an individual, with characteristics particular to their genetic make-up.

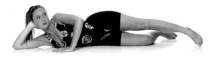

Above: Basic exercises can work wonders.

BODY BRACKETS

Although we come in a variety of shapes and sizes, the human body is cast from one of three basic moulds: ectomorphs; mesomorphs, and endomorphs.

Ectomorphs are usually small- and slender-framed with long limbs, narrow shoulders, hips and joints. They have little muscle or body fat. Mesomorphs have medium to large – but compact – frames with broader shoulders, pelvic girdle and well-developed muscles. Endomorphs are naturally curvaceous, with more body fat than muscle, wider hips, shorter limbs and a lower centre of gravity than the other two body types.

SELF-IMAGE

Very few of us actually see ourselves as we really are. We tend to misjudge our bodies with sweeping claims to fatness, even when we have only a spot of excess flab around our midriff to show for it. And although it sounds amazing, the way we behave in everyday life (and think others see us) often tallies with our self-image. It's a vicious circle: we think that we don't measure up to the standard beauty ideal so our self-esteem dips, often so low that we feel that we will never have a better body. This in turn causes self-confidence to plummet further, we feel even worse, and so the vicious circle continues…

Taking control of your self-image brings enormous bonuses. And the faster you can do this, the greater the rewards, as speedy results boost your confidence more quickly. But before you undertake a scheme to get into better shape, you must work on your positive thinking: realize your potential by deciding on

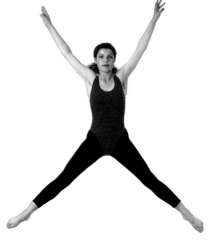

Above: Taking control of your self-image will boost your confidence – and leave you jumping for joy.

(and accepting) your body model, then use this as your goal. Forget conventional beauty ideals – you don't have to have mile-long legs to have a dynamite figure; what you already have, your basic shape, is great. It just needs perfecting, and that is something that everyone can do.

Left: Regular exercise tunes the body and wakens the mind to a lively and positive outlook on life, and you'll soon notice the enormous benefits it brings.

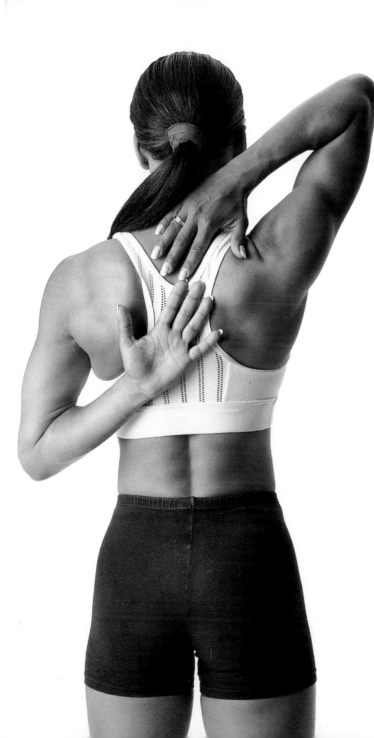

GOOD POSTURE

It sounds like some pointless exercise from your schooldays, but there is real wisdom in the old dictum "head up, shoulders back, bottom in". The difference that good posture makes to the look of our bodies is enormous, mainly because when we are standing properly our abdominal muscles are in their correct supporting role and the whole body is aligned so it looks leaner and taller. Good posture is also helpful to our mental and physical health; alternative therapies such as the Alexander Technique are based on the principle of correct posture because it can ease back pain, stress, and headaches.

Posture Exercise Stand in front of a mirror and see what these exercises do for the shape of your body:
1 Do this exercise facing yourself first, then turn so you are sideways on:
■ Lift your head and lengthen your spine.
■ Tuck in your chin and your bottom.
■ Bring your shoulders back and down.
2 Now stand with your legs slightly apart.
■ Check that your weight is evenly spread.
■ Keep your shoulders and hips level and your weight balanced between the heel and ball of each foot.

Left: Get into the good posture habit.

Below: A flexible body is a fit body.

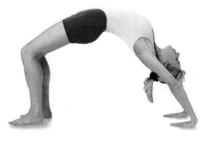

Trouble Spots

Very few people are able to say that they are totally happy with their bodies. Perceived "flaws" can be improved or disguised, but as anyone who has ever tried (and failed) to move the fat that sits on strategic points such as hips, thighs, stomach, and buttocks knows, it is easier to hide the flaws than to tackle them. Trouble spots such as these are notoriously stubborn to shift, but it is possible to alter your outline with a combination of diet and exercise.

COMMON PROBLEMS

Any of the following complaints can be discouraging, but don't despair – just remember every problem has a solution.

Slack stomachs Stomachs become flabby when the abdominal muscles slacken; this usually happens through lack of exercise. Your abdomen extends from just under the bustline to the groin, and it is packed with muscles that criss-cross to form a wall to hold the abdominal contents in place. Exercise is not the only way to keep your stomach flat though: weight is also an important factor and the long-term answer is diet and exercise.

Thunder thighs Thighs are a great source of discontent, whether it is because they are too flabby, muscular, or skinny. You inherit the basic shape of your thighs, but that does not necessarily mean that you were born with the excess fat that may now be covering them. Thigh size and tone can be altered with the right diet, correct body care and regular exercise. Sports such as cycling, skiing, tennis, squash, and riding will tone your thighs, as will weight training.

Large bottoms There are three large muscles in our buttocks: *gluteus maximus, medius,* and *minimus.* These create the shape, but not the size, of our rear ends. It is the tone of these muscles and the fatty tissue around them that gives us the bottoms we have. The good news is that buttock muscles respond well to exercise, which means that any effort you put in will be rewarded quickly. Locomotive exercises – such as fast walking, running, and jogging – are good bottom trimmers.

Slack upper arms Our arms do not change shape much during our lives, unless we lose or gain a lot of weight. Muscle tone is the most common problem, but exercise and specific weight training will tone and shape flabby arms.

Droopy breasts Breast shape and size change when our weight swings dramatically, or during pregnancy, when breast-feeding, or if taking oral contraceptives. Gravity slackens breast tone, and because the breasts are supported by suspensory ligaments and not muscle, you cannot reverse lost tone. Exercising the pectoral muscles beneath your armpits will give your breasts a firmer base and more uplift.

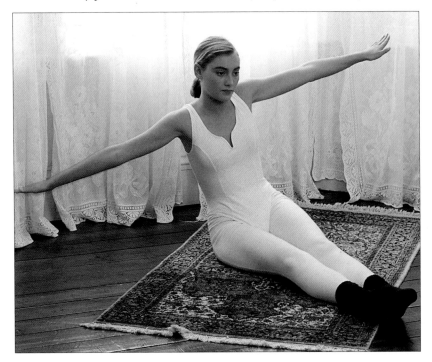

Left: Shape your thighs in a spare 10 minutes. Sit on the floor with your legs out in front of you. Roll sideways on your bottom – go right over on to your outer thigh and then roll right over to the other thigh. Repeat 20 times.

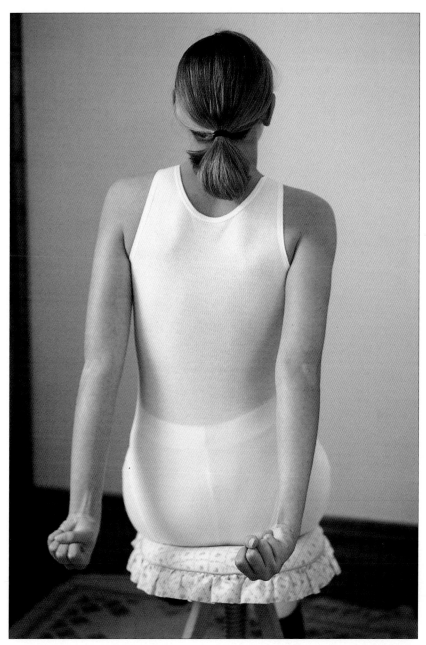

Thick ankles Slender ankles that seem set to snap with every step are a great asset. If you are not blessed with these, or if your ankles tend to become stiff and puffy from fluid retention, you need to master the art of deception and brush up on some ankle improving exercises.

Assess the flexibility of your ankles by sitting on a chair with your feet on the floor and, while keeping your heel down pull your foot up as far as it will go: if the distance between your foot and the floor measures 12–15 cm/5–6 in your joint flexibility is good; if it measures between 10–12 cm/4–5 in it is fair; and if it is less than that, your joint flexibility is poor.

Below: Whenever you remember, move your ankles around clockwise 10 times, then anti-clockwise 10 times.

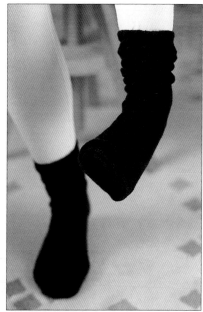

Left: Even flabby arms can be toned up.

Facial Exercises: A Quick Freshener and Toner

Tension shows in your face and makes your features look drawn and your expressions rather set. A good laugh is the best way to relax a tense face, but this exercise routine also helps to liberate and tone the key muscles quickly; try it when you are in the bath – not in your car at the traffic lights.

Tip

Using the backs of your hands alternately, pat the area beneath your chin, using a quick, stroking-like movement. Do this for a few minutes every day to firm up slack skin and help get rid of a double chin.
To firm up slack cheek muscles, fill your mouth with as much water as possible and hold it there for as long as you can to exercise your muscles: the water pressure does all the work.

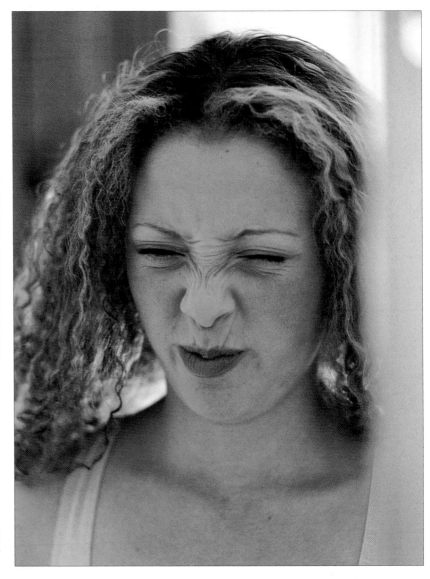

1 Scrunch up your whole face for a few seconds so that your nose is wrinkled, your forehead furrowed, and your eyes and mouth are tightly closed.

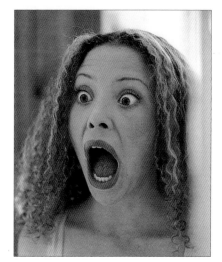

2 Do the opposite: open your mouth and eyes as wide as you can (as if you are silently screaming) to release the tension in your throat muscles.

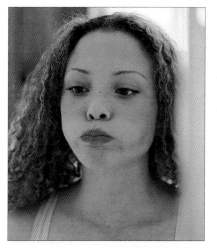

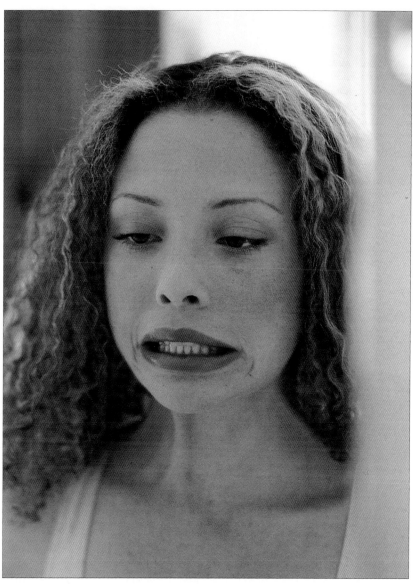

3 Close your mouth again, purse your lips, and push your mouth up first to the left, then to the right.

4 Grin – as if from ear to ear – and open your eyes wide again. Relax your eyes but hold and repeat the grin; this time, tuck your chin well in, until you can feel your neck muscles tighten. Relax and repeat once more.

The General Exercises

WARM-UP EXERCISES

Warm-up exercises gently ease your body into increased activity. The movements should be slow and rhythmical, not sharp and jerky. As well as the exercise below, you could also spend two minutes running up and down the stairs, walking briskly or cycling.

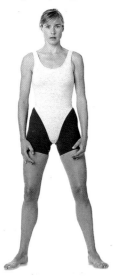

1 Stand with your feet fairly wide apart, and lean forwards slightly from the hips, keeping your chest lifted and your back straight.

Tip

Your body cannot "store" fitness, so keep your routine flexible and easy to maintain. A basic exercise plan done regularly will get better results than an intense work-out done only twice and then abandoned.

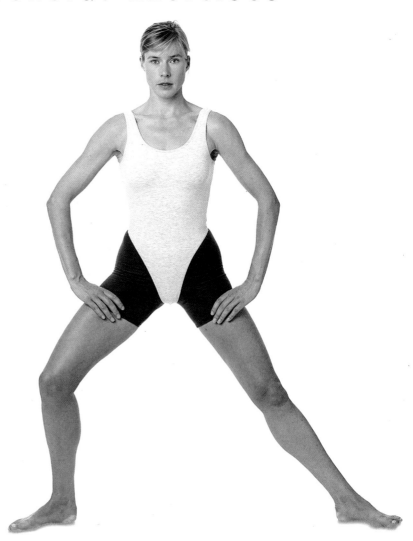

2 Gently rotate and bend your left leg out from the hip until your knee is directly over your left foot and pointing in the same direction. Keep your right leg straight and your right foot pressed into the floor. You should feel a comfortable stretch in the inner thigh; if not, place your legs further apart. Repeat 5 times, holding the position for 5 seconds; swap leg positions and repeat.

CHEST MUSCLES: PRESS-UPS

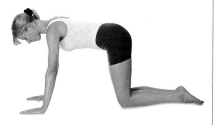

1 Place yourself on all fours with your knees directly under your hips, your hands beneath your shoulders with your fingers pointing forwards, and your palms flat. Keep your back straight – that is, parallel with the ceiling – all the time. Achieve this by pulling your stomach in and tucking in your pelvis.

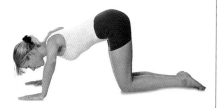

2 Steadily lower yourself – nose first – towards the floor ...

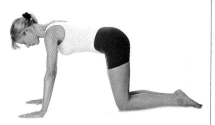

3 ... then raise yourself slowly back to the starting position, breathing in steadily as you go. Repeat 20 times.

UPPER BACK MUSCLES: LYING FLIES

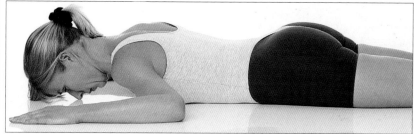

1 Lie on your front on the floor with your hips pressed down. Try to keep your body relaxed. Rest your forehead on the floor, and keep your arms stretched out on each side at right angles to your body, with your elbows bent.

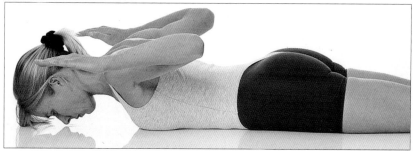

2 Still keeping your elbows bent, steadily lift both arms, making sure they are parallel to the floor. Raise them slowly, and keep them at the same level.

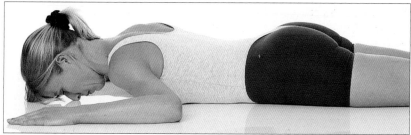

3 Lower both your arms to the floor once again. Make sure you don't pull your elbows back; keep them in line with your shoulders and keep your hips and feet in contact with the floor all the time. Repeat 20 times.

ABDOMINAL MUSCLES

When you do these exercises, keep your lower back pressed into the floor throughout and work slowly, with total control. In the Upper Abdominals exercise, lift your head and shoulders as one unit, never separately; roll up from the top of your head; if it helps, imagine you are holding a peach between your chin and your chest and try to keep this gap constant throughout. Make sure you keep your facial muscles loose and relaxed all the time.

LOWER ABDOMINALS: REVERSE CURLS

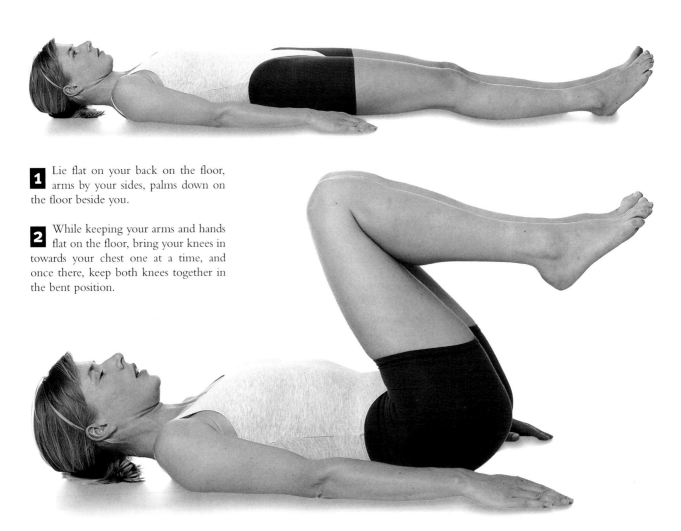

1 Lie flat on your back on the floor, arms by your sides, palms down on the floor beside you.

2 While keeping your arms and hands flat on the floor, bring your knees in towards your chest one at a time, and once there, keep both knees together in the bent position.

3 Breathe in and, keeping your spine firmly pressed into the floor, pull in your abdominal muscles while at the same time curling up your coccyx (tail bone) to bring your knees closer to your chest. Keep your feet relaxed throughout. Lower your body to the starting position, exhaling as you go down.

Important note
With all exercise, if you feel any pain or experience anything other than the normal sensation of muscle fatigue, stop exercising. Always work at your own pace and quit if you begin to feel dizzy. Skip exercise altogether if you are ill, or have a virus or a raised temperature.

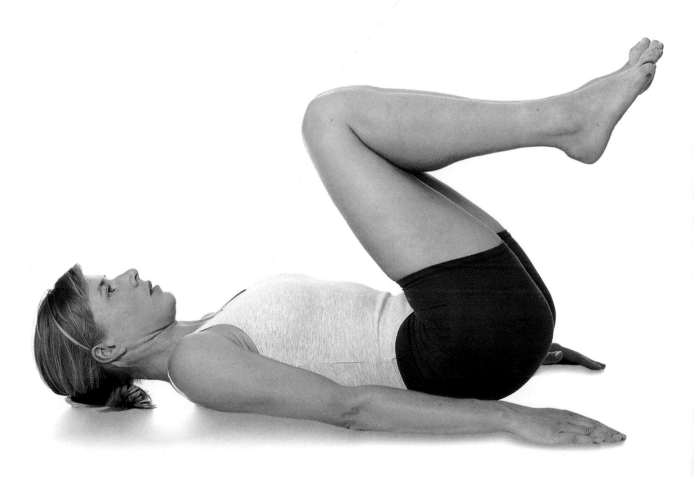

UPPER ABDOMINALS: SIT UPS

1 Lying flat on the floor with your arms by your sides, and your palms down, bend your knees and keep your feet flat on the floor, a little distance apart and in line with your hips.

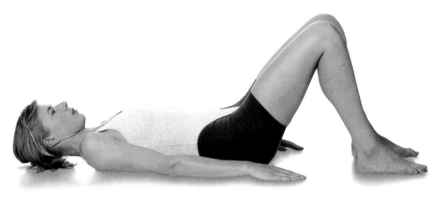

2 Lift your head and shoulders upwards – inhaling as you move up – and push your fingertips towards your knees, keeping your arms straight.

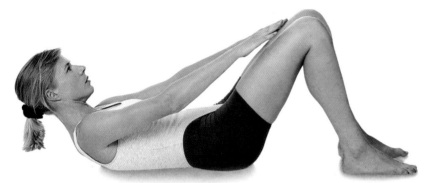

3 Lower your body back to the starting position, breathing out as you go down. When you get to the floor, do not allow yourself a stop to rest but repeat the movement, from Step 1.

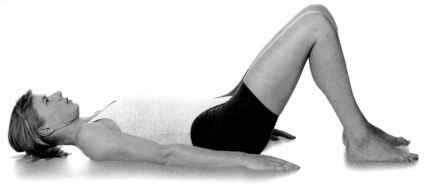

LEG MUSCLES: SQUATS

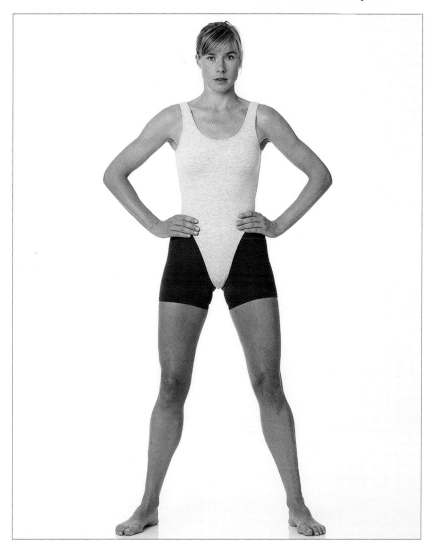

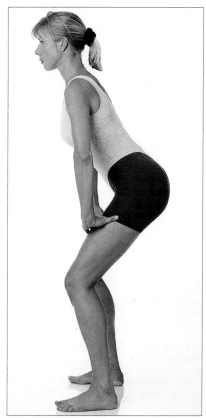

2 Resting your hands on the front of your thighs and keeping your arms straight, steadily bend your legs to a squatting position, breathing out slowly as you go down.

3 Then, inhale as you rise steadily back to the starting position. When you do this exercise, it is important to keep your back straight and your knees flexible. Don't let your knees bend further forward than your toes.

1 Stand up straight with your feet a little further apart than shoulder-width. If you stand on tiptoe, this exercise will tone your calf muscles and your quadriceps (the muscles on the front of your thighs); if you angle your toes slightly outwards while on tiptoe, it will benefit your inner thighs.

Index

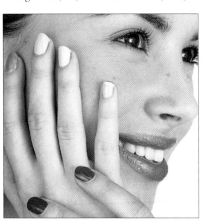

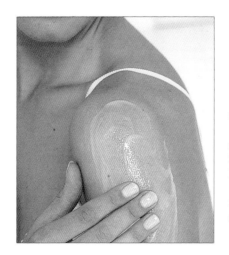

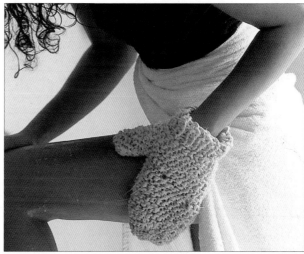

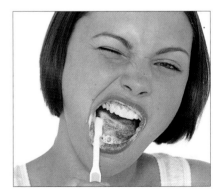